HERBAL HANDBOOK

DEEPAK CHOPRA

and

DAVID SIMON

RIDER

LONDON · SYDNEY · AUCKLAND · JOHANNESBURG

1 3 5 7 9 10 8 6 4 2

First Published in 2000 by Three Rivers Press,
an imprint of Crown Publishing Group, Random House Inc., USA
This edition published in 2000 by Rider,
an imprint of Ebury Press, Random House,
20 Vauxhall Bridge Road, London SW1V 2SA
www.randomhouse.co.uk

The Random House Group Limited supports The Forest Stewardship Council (FSC®), the leading international forest certification organisation. Our books carrying the FSC label are printed on FSC® certified paper. FSC is the only forest certification scheme endorsed by the leading environmental organisations, including Greenpeace. Our paper procurement policy can be found at www.randomhouse.co.uk/environment

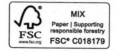

The Random House Group Limited Reg. No. 954009

Design by LYNNE AMFT

Printed and bound in Great Britain by Clays Ltd, St Ives PLC

A CIP catalogue record for this book
is available from the British Library

ISBN 0-7126-0167-8

This book gives non-specific, general advice and should not be relied on as a substitute for proper medical consultation. The author and publisher cannot accept responsibility for illness arising out of the failure to seek medical advice from a doctor.

To the staff members of the Chopra Center for
Well Being who on a daily basis devote themselves to
meeting the physical, emotional, and spiritual needs
of our guests and patients;

To the team members of MyPotential.com,
who support the vision of empowering people to live
a more fulfilling life;

and

To all loving souls on this planet who are committed
to healing themselves and the world.

ACKNOWLEDGMENTS

We'd like to acknowledge our family and friends who have supported the birth and development of this book:

Pamela, Max, and Sara Simon;

Rita Chopra, Gautama Chopra,
Mallika Chopra Mandal, and Sumant Mandal;

Peter Guzzardi;

Muriel Nellis and Jane Roberts;

and

James Nocito, for his beautiful artwork.

OTHER BOOKS BY DEEPAK CHOPRA

Creating Health

Return of the Rishi

Quantum Healing

Perfect Health

Unconditional Life

Ageless Body, Timeless Mind

Perfect Weight

Perfect Digestion

Journey into Healing

Creating Affluence

*The Seven Spiritual Laws of
  Success*

The Return of Merlin

Boundless Energy

Restful Sleep

The Way of the Wizard

Overcoming Addictions

Raid on the Inarticulate

The Path to Love

*The Seven Spiritual Laws
  for Parents*

The Love Poems of Rumi
(edited by Deepak Chopra; translated by
Deepak Chopra and Fereydoun Kia)

Healing the Heart

Everyday Immortality

The Lords of the Light

On the Shores of Eternity

How to Know God

CHOPRA CENTRE BOOKS BY DAVID SIMON

The Wisdom of Healing

The Chopra Centre Cookbook
(with Ginna Bell Bragg)

WEB SITES

If you have enjoyed this book and wish to learn more about ways to enhance your physical, emotional, and spiritual well being, visit our new Web site:

www.MyPotential.com

For more information about programs and courses offered through the Chopra Center for Well Being, visit our Web site:

www.Chopra.com

CONTENTS

1

The Herbal Renaissance

The Lord created medicines out of the earth, and the wise do not reject them.

—BOOK OF SIRACH 38:4

We are witnessing an unprecedented resurgence in natural healing. The search for holistic approaches to enhance health is permeating every aspect of our culture and society. Why is there such an explosive interest in natural medicine? It is certainly not for lack of success from our scientific approach to illness. Major advances in physiology, biochemistry, pharmacology, and genetics have exponentially expanded our understanding of disease, and we have developed previously unimaginable new ways to diagnose and treat the afflictions of humanity. Within the last fifty years we have eradicated smallpox, minimized the risk of many life-threatening childhood diseases, performed sophisticated brain surgery, and transplanted organs. In view of these obvious successes of our modern medical system, we might imagine that the status of the institutions of medicine would be at an all-time high. And yet we know there is pervasive dissatisfaction and frustration with our health care. How can we explain this paradox?

1

It is the nature of life to strive continually for more evolutionary solutions to the endless challenges that arise. In this information age, every intelligent person has access to a vast body of facts and opinions on any subject of interest. People facing health concerns no longer depend solely upon their physicians for advice and information on the management of their illness. Whether or not you have a health-care background, you have unprecedented opportunities to learn about your problem. Through the Internet, books, journals, newsletters, and support groups, more and more people are formulating their own view of their illness and how they want to approach it. Patients are no longer passive and are not inclined to be as patient as they once were. There is a powerful movement of self-empowerment and consumerism in the world today that grew in part out of the sixties mindset of challenging authority. Thalidomide, DES, Fen-Phen, and other highly publicized drug recalls over the past generation have dampened our unbridled enthusiasm for consuming every new pharmaceutical product as the shortest distance between sickness and health. With expanding information on the role of diet, stress, and activity on health and disease, many people are asking these new questions of their health providers: *What should I be eating to help my body heal? How can I better manage my stress? Is there a role for nutritional supplements in the treatment of my condition?*

Such questions reflect a deeper one, which we hear each day at the Chopra Center for Well Being: *What more can I do to be an active partner in my healing process?* Unfortunately, most of our medical colleagues are ill-prepared to answer these questions, and often discourage their patients from asking them, directly or indirectly. Consequently, more people are seeking alternative sources of information. The now well-known report of Dr. David Eisenberg showed that more than two in five Americans sought out "unconventional" medical treatment in 1997, while other studies have put the number at closer to one in two.[1, 2]

What needs are being fulfilled by these unorthodox modalities? In our experience at the Chopra Center, most people have not rejected medical care; they simply want to explore other, less toxic alternatives before resorting to a potent drug or procedure; they want to be more than passive receptacles of physician-prescribed drugs; they want to go beyond compliance to active partnership. It is here that herbal medicine can make a contribution to the well-being of individuals and of our community.

According to Ayurveda, India's ancient medical system, human beings are not merely thinking physical machines frozen in time and space. Rather, we are networks of intelligence in a universe of energy and information. The conscious energy field of the universe organizes into forms and phenomena spanning the entire range from galaxies to subatomic particles. Somewhere in between are human beings, with their physical, emotional, psychological, and spiritual layers. We are in constant and dynamic exchange with our environment through our breathing, eating, eliminating, perceptions, and interpretations. It is an illusion of our senses that our boundaries end abruptly at the surface of our skin.

Within this framework, health is more than the mere absence of a laboratory abnormality; it is the dynamic integration of environment, body, mind, and spirit. Herbal medicine offers a gentle approach to enhance this integration, particularly when the imbalance has not gone too far. Healing plants allow us to reconnect with our environment, accessing the power of nature as our ancestors have done since antiquity. Herbs can help us normalize disturbed physiological functions including digestion, elimination and sleep. They can help restore weakened immunity, settle a turbulent mind and promote detoxification and rejuvenation. Plants provide us expanded and diverse options to synthesized drugs, but they do not replace the appropriate use of pharmaceuticals.

We wouldn't use a jackhammer to knock a nail into a wall, nor would we expect to remove the nail with a tweezers. There is an appropriate tool for every job, and this is certainly true for medicines. In our earlier days as medical doctors, we would at times prescribe a medication, simply because we did not have any other tools in our toolbox. If we saw someone with annoying migraines, we would prescribe a headache medicine. If we believed that a patient was suffering with mild depression, we would prescribe an antidepressant. Difficulty sleeping? Chronic back pain? Indigestion? We could justify prescribing a pharmacological agent for just about any problem you might have.

When we began seriously and systematically to use holistic approaches, we saw people with conditions in which subtler, natural options were more effective, with fewer side effects, than any medication we could offer.

One of David's first experiences with natural medicine was with a woman with migraine headaches who had not responded to treatment for over a year. Despite a trial of every known headache drug, her discomfort persisted, creating frustration for the patient and her doctors, who received regular calls from the emergency room announcing her arrival. Finally, out of desperation, she was taught a simple meditation technique, instructed to make minor changes in her diet, and she was prescribed an herbal tea made of feverfew. After just a few weeks she related a major improvement in her headache pattern, and within six months no longer required medical care for what had been a lifelong condition. Deepak vividly recalls one of his early cases in which he prescribed herbal aromatherapy for a woman with life-threatening heart irregularities. She was taught to associate the herbal scent with a healing meditation technique and was eventually able to eliminate her need for medication, to the astonishment of her cardiologist. The plural of anecdote is not science, but even doctors can be impressed by their personal experiences. We are increasingly reassured by the growing body of scientific literature demonstrating the measurable benefits of herbal remedies, which we see every day at the Chopra Center.

On the other hand, people sometimes have unrealistic expectations of herbs. Resorting to a blend of wishful thinking and denial, women with abnormal mammograms, smokers with problematic chest X-rays, and overweight people with dangerously elevated blood sugars may go on quests to find the "magical" herb that will cause their physical problem to evaporate, preferably without any other lifestyle change. With these patients, we have learned that compassionate, honest education is the key to enlisting their choice of a course that is realistic and likely to succeed. Herbs can add tremendous value in these circumstances, but they are not a substitute for appropriate medical care.

An herbal medicine can be a powerful ingredient in a holistic health program, but it should not be expected to carry the entire healing responsibility. Herbs can help support, nourish, and balance the physiology, and they can help detoxify and replenish, but although they can play an important role, herbs should not, by themselves, be expected to eradicate metastatic cancer, cure infertility, or reverse an inherited degenerative disease. Our goal in this book is to honor plant-based medicines for their contribution to our health without over- or underestimating their value. With this approach, we believe we will see a greater interest in, and acceptance of, these powerful, ancient healing substances.

The Antidote to Anguish and Alienation

In our growing mastery of the world, we may forget that there is a profound underlying intelligence that expresses itself in nature. Many people living in urban centers spend days, weeks, and months without the opportunity to immerse themselves in a natural environment. Driving through rush-hour traffic to work in an office without access to fresh air alienates us from our environment and ultimately from ourselves. Fast-food meals and commercial entertainment provide few reminders that we ourselves are magnificent expressions of Mother Nature. We believe that deep in our evolutionary soul we long for a sense of connection to our environment. Our resurgent fascination with herbs may nurture that part of our spirit that is calling for a simpler life and a more innocent time when we felt closer to the natural world. Perhaps we are enamored with herbal medicines because it is in our nature to use the plants in our environment to balance and heal us. To this end, we hope *The Chopra Center Herbal Handbook* provides valuable guidance on your journey to well-being.

2

A Brief Tour through Herbal History

Once upon a time, a small, apelike creature pulled itself up on two legs to get a better view of its environment. Over the next several million years, its brain got bigger while its hair got thinner, until about 100,000 years ago a tool-using, language-creating being evolved that anthropologists now call human. While sampling their surroundings, human beings developed an unwritten roster of which plants in their environment tasted good, tasted bad, made them feel better, or made them sick. This knowledge of vegetative power, passed down from generation to generation, was collected to answer the perennial questions that all of us face at times: How can I fulfill my hunger? How can I relieve my suffering? How can I maintain my vitality?

Long before our beginning as human beings, we were inextricably interwoven with the plant kingdom. We cannot imagine a world without green things, because we could not exist without plants. From the time that plants and animals

7

took their first separate evolutionary steps, we have remained interdependent. Without the alchemy that plants perform of transforming light into sugar and oxygen, animals could not have arisen or survived. We owe our very existence to the herbal kingdom, although most of us rarely even consider the contribution of herbs to our well-being. Although we supply carbon dioxide for their consumption, our growing exploitation of the natural environment leaves us in deepening debt to the generous greenery that has sustained the animal world for millions of years. One of our hopes in writing this book is to add to the growing chorus of voices striving to alert humanity to the recklessly dangerous self-destructive path that decimating our natural habitats heralds. Immense untapped healing wisdom lives in the plants of our planet, and it is both our responsibility and our birthright to honor the gifts they offer. Let's spend a few moments looking at the important role that healing plants have played in our lives since the dawn of humankind.

In the Beginning

The evolution of herbal medicine is a fascinating story. As every parent experiences firsthand, infant human beings have a tendency to put everything into their mouths. We suspect that early humans had a similar propensity, sampling every fruit, flower, leaf, bark, and root, looking for sources of nourishment. At times they discovered powerful medicines, and at other times powerful poisons. Often the same plant could be both, depending upon the dosage and part ingested. A few leaves of foxglove infused into a tea could strengthen the heart, while a more potent brew could stop it altogether, after first causing vomiting and turning one's vision green. Drops of sap from an unripe poppy could soothe a crampy digestive tract and relieve the pain of a wound, but too much would lead to constipation, lethargy, and even death. A decoction of senna pods might induce a complete bowel evacuation, but a few too many leaves could empty a person to the point of dehydration. Some plants had powerful actions, while others were subtler. After discovering the effect of a particular plant, efforts to define the most potent components would follow, be it the leaf, root, or berry. Herbal knowledge advanced through trial and error, without the benefit of animal testing, but almost certainly with the benefit of animal observation. Many wild animals, from birds to gorillas, seek out specific plants when they are feeling under the weather. Attentive hunters may have noticed the bear chewing long pepper after her fray with a venomous viper, or a wolf eating ipecac to induce vomiting after consuming a poisonous lizard, and subsequently investigated their medicinal properties.

As tribes became more proficient in meeting their basic survival needs, specialized roles could be supported, the first of which was that of the medicine person. In addition to knowledge about the spirit world, the tribal healer developed a repertoire of secret healing substances that was jealously guarded, selectively handed down to suitably prepared initiates. Native cultures on every continent developed healing traditions replete with medicines derived from nature's pharmacy. Although the herbal traditions of Africa may be older, the recording of medicinal substances was first achieved in Asia.

Over 4,500 years ago the Chinese emperor Shen Nung cataloged a compendium of medicinal herbs. At about the same time, Indus Valley healers organized the body of knowledge that has come to be known as Ayurveda. In both of these ancient cultures, healing herbs and the knowledge of how to use them were held to be of divine origin. In their compassion for the suffering of humanity, the gods bestowed their wisdom on the humble healing sages of antiquity, who transmitted it to their students.

In Ayurveda, the timeless healing system from India, the ascetic sage Bhardwaja went to Lord Indra to learn how human beings could live long, happy lives. Bhardwaja imparted this knowledge to Atreya, who handed it to Agnivesa, the first to write it down. The subsequent expansion by Charaka, a later disciple in the school of Atreya, is still available today and remains one of the classic texts of Ayurveda, describing almost four hundred medicinal herbs. One of Atreya's eminent students, Jivaka, is said to have passed his final exam by returning empty-handed after receiving instructions to bring back all useless plants from the kingdom. With this response he demonstrated the essential principle of Ayurveda—that all things have healing potential.

Closer to home, the Egyptian school of medicine founded in Alexandria three hundred years before the birth of Christ is believed to have accumulated a substantial body of medical knowledge. Unfortunately, we'll never know for sure, since all the medical texts, along with 700,000 other books, were burned by religious fanatics in the fourth century A.D. The Greek system of medicine, established at about the same time as the Alexandrian school, fared somewhat better. Hippocrates, in his *Materia Medica,* carefully described many herbal medicines still prized today, including poppy, rosemary, sage, and mugwort. Several hundred years later, in the first century A.D., another Greek physician, Dioscorides, compiled *De Materia Medica.* In his work, the physician to Emperor Nero described the use of over five hundred healing herbs. This work remained the standard text of the medical arts through the Middle Ages.

The discovery of the New World by European explorers can largely be attributed to the importance of herbal medicine. Five hundred years ago the great Western European powers felt exploited by the merchants trafficking in herbs and spices from the Far East. Finding a shortcut to the botanical riches of India was the primary goal of Columbus when he sailed west at the end of the fifteenth century. The unanticipated interruption of his trip between Europe and Asia by the American continent opened a new chapter in the history of the world and medicine.

The New World unveiled a bounty of natural resources, including tens of thousands of unique botanicals. Europeans encountered Native American cultures that possessed rich and reliable knowledge of the medicinal value of hundreds of indigenous plants. Early settlers in the seventeenth and eighteenth centuries experienced the healing potency of many native plants that remain household words today. Ginger, goldenseal, black cohosh, sassafras, ginseng, and angelica are just a few of the original flora that were known to aboriginal Americans and valued as healing substances. Efforts to systematically catalog the natural pharmacy of America were unfortunately neglected until many of the traditional healing cultures had been destroyed. The contribution of indigenous American medicine was finally recognized by the renowned Philadelphia physician Benjamin Rush, who thus empowered other early-nineteenth-century doctors to compile guides to Native American plant lore. The practice of medicine in nineteenth-century America blended a rich botanical pharmacy with an expanding choice of chemically derived substances at a time when the division between natural and scientific medicine had not yet been established.

Medicine in the Scientific Age

The medical pharmacopoeia two hundred years ago was a primarily a botanical compendium; not until the early 1800s were the first chemically derived drugs developed. One of the earliest efforts was that of F. W. A. Sertürner, who extracted white crystals from opium, which, when given to dogs, put them to sleep. He called this powder morphine, after Morpheus, the Greek god of dreams. With the development of more-sophisticated chemical methods, alkaloids from other powerful plants were distilled, including cocaine from coca leaves and quinine from the cinchona tree. As more purified and concentrated derivatives of plants became available, the importance of the original botanical sources faded into the background. The prioritization of synthesized drugs over natural sources became so complete that modern students at Western medical universities receive no formal training in the use of botanicals. Today's physicians apply the term "medicine" solely to compounds created by a pharmaceutical company and ingested in the form of a tablet or capsule. The idea that an infusion, tea, or tincture derived from an herb can be a therapeutic substance is a foreign concept to most Western medical doctors.

The scientific age has brought us unparalleled prosperity. The application of modern physics and chemistry principles has enabled human beings to survive and thrive in an almost unlimited range of environments. With cellular telephones, fax machines, lightweight plastics, and synthetic fibers we are capable of exploring and communicating from outer space and the depths of the oceans. Applying scientific principles to medicine has led to remarkable diagnostic and therapeutic discoveries that have improved the quality and length of our lives. Our ability to treat acute illnesses is unprecedented in the history of humanity. However, our exclusive reliance upon drugs in the treatment of illness has also led to antibiotic-resistant bacteria and hundreds of thousands of serious annual medical complications resulting from the overuse or misuse of pharmacological agents.

In our quest to synthesize new and more-powerful pharmaceuticals, the medical community has forgotten the important role that medicinal plants continue to play. Of the 150 most popular pharmaceutical products sold today, over eighty contain active ingredients derived from natural sources. From morphine to Metamucil, from quinine to camphor, from aspirin to atropine, many of our modern medicines are rooted in substances with roots. Recently we have been reminded of the importance of plant sources of drugs with the discovery of taxol, the powerful chemotherapy agent derived from the Pacific yew tree. This was the result of a concerted National Cancer Institute program in which more than thirty thousand plants were screened for medicinal activity.[1] Other important cancer-fighting drugs have been derived from botanical sources, including vincristine and vinblastine, from the Madagascan periwinkle, and etoposide, a powerful chemotherapy agent from the May apple plant.

Only about 2 percent of the more than 250,000 species of higher plants have been carefully evaluated for medicinal activity. One company, Shaman Pharmaceuticals, has used anthropological information about healing substances to test plants for medicinal activity. In a review of over two hundred plants that are used to fight infectious diseases in traditional healing systems, they found that over 60 percent showed some activity against viruses growing in a laboratory.[2] The potential for deriving unique and powerful medicines from the vegetable kingdom is immense, but with deforestation of our rain forests occurring at a rate of over 34,000 square miles each year, we are at continuous risk of losing valuable and irreplaceable healing plants. For our health and the health of our ecology, we need to regain the reverence for the plant kingdom that was expressed in an ancient Vedic hymn:

> *You Herbs, born at the birth of*
> *time*
> *More ancient than the gods*
> *themselves.*
> *O Plants, with this hymn I sing*
> *to you*
> *Our mothers and our gods.*

The Economics of Nature

Herbal medicine has never left us, although for most of the last generation she has been in hibernation. In the United States we have not established a place for herbs in our therapeutic armamentarium, so we have relegated them to the same category as food. The U.S. Food and Drug Administration (FDA) requires any substance purported to have therapeutic value to go through a safety and efficacy process that usually costs hundreds of millions of dollars. Since most herbal products use unprocessed or minimally processed plant material, it is essentially impossible to get an exclusive patent on a medicinal herb. Therefore it is not financially feasible for a pharmaceutical company to invest the money necessary to obtain FDA approval. The only other option has been to label herbs as dietary supplements, which means that no specific therapeutic claims can be made for them. This approach has led to very little regulated or reliable information on how to use herbal medicines safely and rationally. Unfortunately, owing to the lack of information on herbs provided to physicians in training at Western medical colleges, the role of herbs has remained marginal.

This does not mean that the American public has neglected medicinal herbs. Indeed, recent estimates are that one in three Americans spends more than fifty dollars per year on herbs, adding up to a collective value of over $3 billion in 1996.[3] Just one year later the estimate rose to over $5 billion.[4] Over $90 million is spent on *Gingko biloba* alone, and with recent studies confirming its efficacy in Alzheimer's disease, gingko's usage will undoubtedly expand even further.[5] Reports confirming the value of St. John's wort for depression will surely increase its popularity above and beyond the nearly fifty million dollars spent on it in 1997.[6]

In Europe, unlike America, herbs have held a more acceptable status among the mainstream medical establishment. Herbal products stand side by side with prescription drugs in European pharmacies and are classified as medicines. About 1,400 herbal substances are available in the European community, with 1996 sales amounting to more than $7 billion. In the field of herbology, Germany stands out as the most progressive Western country, with an estimated 30 percent of all botanical medicines prescribed by medical doctors, and more than three out of four doctors routinely prescribing herbs in their practice. The American Botanical Council has recently published the English translation of the German Commission E Monographs, which is a compilation of the medicinal value of almost four hundred herbs.[7] The commission, founded by the German Federal Health Agency, reviewed information from scientific and traditional sources to reach its findings on the safety and efficacy of these herbal products. The result of this integrative approach is that the polarity between mainstream and alternative medicine has diminished, and mainstream medical doctors have the opportunity to witness the benefits of herbal medicine firsthand. Our hope is that as our collective awareness of the value of nature's pharmacy rises in America, our health-care system will remember that the purpose of medicine is to relieve suffering, and that this purpose transcends all other concerns. Fortunately there are recent signs that we are moving in this direction. A recent report in the *Journal of the American Medical Association* found that almost two out of three medical schools are now offering some type of introductory course in complementary and alternative medicine.[8] As credible information on the value of herbal medicine becomes available, we can hope to see a continuation of this trend and the dissolving of the artificial boundary between "orthodox/allopathic" and "holistic/alternative." This book is dedicated to moving us a few steps closer to the integrated approach to life and health that, as understood by Jivaka and King Solomon, recognizes that "to every thing there is a season, and a time to every purpose under heaven." Surely there is a time and purpose for the abundant healing resources from our herbal kingdom.

3

Holistically Herbal

The relief of suffering is a noble goal. In pursuit of this end, herbal medicines can play an important role. However, we are not proponents of herbal allopathy. One of the most frequent complaints we hear about Western medicine is that it is too symptom-oriented. If you have indigestion, your doctor can prescribe an antacid or an H_2 receptor blocker. For your arthritis there's an anti-inflammatory medicine. There are laxatives for your constipation, sleeping pills for your insomnia, and muscle relaxants for your back strain. Most of these pharmaceuticals provide temporary symptomatic relief, but have limited impact on the basic cause of the illness. Mahatma Gandhi once lamented that the problem with Western medicine is that it is *too* effective. A person can eat a meal of junk food devoid of nutritional value, develop terrible indigestion, and then take a couple of antacid tablets. Within a few minutes the condition is relieved without the person having to pay any consequences for his choices. The medications short-circuit Mother Nature's feedback loop, and as a result there is little motivation to change behavior.

It is possible to use herbal medicines in a similar way. If your bowels are sluggish, you can take some *Cascara sagrada*. For your migraine headaches there is feverfew. Feeling a little anxious? Try some kava. These days there are almost as many herbal approaches to common health concerns as there are pharmacological ones. We often see people who believe they are following a natural health-enhancing program because they are taking a host of herbs and nutritional supplements. Although herbs can provide value as symptomatic medicines, they are much more powerful when used as part of a holistic healing program. Rather than simply taking valerian to help you sleep at night, look at the underlying issues that are keeping you awake. Instead of automatically resorting to amalaki or licorice for your heartburn, explore your diet and lifestyle for areas of improvement that may make the need for an acid-neutralizing substance unnecessary.

Years ago we heard a renowned Ayurvedic doctor say that herbs are to healing as an inheritance is to success. If children are truly worthy, no inheritance is necessary, because they will be capable of generating their own success. Alternatively, if the children are unworthy of the inheritance, no amount of money will be of much value to them, as they are likely to squander their resources. In an analogous way, if a person is living a balanced life, herbal medicines provide health-promoting advantages, but if a person is not living a balanced life, an herb alone will not be able to compensate fully for poor diet, lack of exercise, or a toxic lifestyle. The gifts from nature's garden are of tremendous value, but they are not a substitute for a life in balance. Let's look at how we can use herbs in conjunction with basic components of a healthy lifestyle to create the highest level of well-being.

Eat Healthy

According to Ayurveda, food is our best medicine, for the physical body is essentially DNA wrapped in food. What we eat and how we eat it determines our health and vitality. Before adding herbal supplements, look at your diet and make certain that it is balanced and delicious. To ensure that your meals are nourishing and appetizing, become familiar with the "Six Tastes" approach. Everything we can ingest through our mouth can be classified according to one or more of six primary tastes: sweet, sour, salty, pungent, bitter, or astringent. *Sweet* taste characterizes foods that are sources of carbohydrates, protein, or fat. Pasta, bread, dairy, rice, grains, fish and meat are considered sweet. We consume the *sour* taste, which is due to natural organic acids, in the form of citrus fruits, berries, and tomatoes. Fermented foods, including yogurt, cheese, and vinegar, are also sources of dietary sour. We get the *salty* flavor from table salt, soy sauce, and seafood. The *pungent* taste is carried in onions, garlic, peppers, and many spices, including black pepper, cayenne, thyme, cinnamon, basil, and cloves. Foods with the *bitter* flavor include green leafy vegetables, other green and yellow vegetables, and many bitter herbs such as cilantro, coriander, cumin, dill, and fenugreek. Most medicinal herbs have a predominantly bitter taste. The *astringent* taste creates a sensation of puckering on the

Taste	Function	Common Sources
SWEET	• most nutritive • builds body tissue	sugar, honey, milk, butter, rice, breads, pastas, meats (carbohydrates, fats, proteins)
SOUR	• improves appetite and digestion • promotes digestion	citrus fruits, yogurt, cheese, tomatoes, pickles, vinegar (organic acids)
SALTY	• mildly laxative/sedative • promotes digestion	salt, sauces, salted meats and fish (mineral salts)
PUNGENT	• stimulates digestion • clears congestion	hot peppers, salsa, ginger, radishes, mustard, cloves, horseradish (essential oils)
BITTER	• anti-inflammatory • detoxifying	green leafy vegetables, celery, sprouts, beets, lemon rind (alkaloids, glycosides)
ASTRINGENT	• drying • compacts system	beans, tea, apples, cabbage, pomegranates, cauliflower, dark leafy greens (tannins)

mucous membranes due to the presence of tannic acids. Beans, legumes, cranberries, pomegranate, and green tea are common sources of the astringent taste. If all six tastes are present at each meal, ample calories, protein, vitamins, minerals, and natural, health-promoting plant chemicals will be abundant in your diet.

We can use herbs to ensure that all six tastes are available at each meal. Herbs and spices add flavor and help enhance our appetite and digestion. Bitter and pungent herbs are most useful to stimulate our digestive juices. A ginger apéritif made from equal parts fresh ginger juice, lemon juice, and water, sweetened with a little honey, is a delicious and potent appetite enlivener. If your appetite has been suppressed by recent illness or emotional distress, bitter herbs can stimulate your digestive fire. The classic bitter herb is gentian, a root used in cultures around the world for its detoxifying and appetite-enhancing effect. Fifteen minutes before a meal, mix one-quarter teaspoon of gentian powder with black pepper and allow it to dissolve on your tongue before swallowing the blend. This will start your salivary and gastric juices flowing, enabling you to digest your food more effectively.

Many culinary herbs and spices have both flavor-enhancing and digestive benefits. Basil, cayenne, mustard seeds, oregano, savory, and thyme all supply the pungent taste and strengthen digestion.

Cumin, coriander, fennel, and dill are less intense digestive enhancers, ideal for people who need digestive stimulation but have a tendency toward heartburn and indigestion. If you are inclined toward gas and bloating, try adding bay leaves, cardamom, cinnamon, cloves, mint, or nutmeg to your cooking. The balanced use of culinary herbs and spices can transform a boring meal into a sumptuous feast that is nourishing and digestible.

Eat Consciously

How we eat is as important as *what* we eat. The way we prepare and consume a meal is as essential to its nourishing effects as its composition of carbohydrate, protein, vitamins, and minerals. Trying to make up for food hastily prepared and hurriedly eaten with nutritional supplements doesn't work. Your attention is the most powerful healing force available to you, and eating with awareness can transform your meals from mere refueling into a healing experience. Try paying attention to the following five simple principles, and watch your quality of nourishment rise.

1. *Listen to your appetite.* Eat when you are really hungry and stop when you are full. This means listening to and honoring the signals of your body. When it is mealtime, ask yourself, "Am I really hungry now?" If the answer

is no, wait a while, observing your appetite until you are ready to feed your digestive fire.

2. *Pay attention to what you are eating.* Try not to be doing other things when eating, such as watching television, talking on the phone, driving, or working. Focusing on the sensations, sights, flavors, and smells of your food enhances your digestion and improves your ability to extract nourishment from your meals.

3. *Eat to fulfill your nutritional needs.* You cannot satisfy emotional needs with food. Although you may experience temporary calming of emotional turbulence after eating a piece of cheesecake, the benefits will be short-lived. Address your emotional needs through self-inspection and open and honest communication. Address your nutritional needs through healthy, balanced, lovingly prepared meals.

4. *Favor freshly prepared foods.* To the greatest extent possible, minimize your intake of canned, frozen, leftover, microwaved, and highly processed foods. Take time to choose and prepare vegetables, whole grains, and legumes that are rich in vital energy. For most people, lightly cooked vegetables are easier to digest than raw ones. Fresh fruit and vegetable juices are rich sources of nutrients and a healthy alternative to nutritionally empty sodas.

5. *Honor your mealtimes.* Define a time and space for your meals that allow you to honor the sacred act of metabolizing the energy and information of your environment into the substance of your body. If you are eating in a rush, you are less likely to be discerning about what or how much you consume. Stop eating when you are satiated, rather than when there is nothing left on your plate. Make certain that all six tastes are present at each meal, and you will avoid the tendency to eat more in order to feel satiated.

Eliminate Toxicity

Everything we ingest can be evaluated in terms of whether it provides us with nourishment or toxicity. Look at your environment and see if there are sources of toxicity that you can reduce or eliminate. We may not be able to control directly the concentration of ozone in our atmosphere, but we can eliminate toxic substances from our personal environment. We may not be able to create peace in the Balkans, but we can improve our personal relationships through greater understanding and tolerance. Look at your home and work environments and see how you can transform toxicity into nourishment. Eliminate tobacco, excessive alcohol, and drugs from your life. Release from your heart self-destructive emotions such as resentment, hostility, and regret. Release from your mind limiting beliefs, including self-loathing and prejudice. In the clearing of toxicity from your body, mind, and soul, vitality and well-being will again flow freely.

Herbs can be very helpful in reducing physical toxicity. If you have been overeating or indulging in unhealthy behaviors, simplify your diet and take aloe vera juice internally in a dosage of one ounce twice daily. Ginger tea, made from one teaspoon of grated fresh ginger per pint of hot water, is also helpful in encouraging your body to detoxify. If you are attempting to stop smoking, try sucking on a natural cinnamon stick whenever you have the urge; the sweet spiciness of cinnamon can be a natural substitute for tobacco while satisfying your oral needs. Sucking on clove buds can provide a similar benefit. Short-term use of bitter herbs such as goldenseal, echinacea, and neem can be helpful in clearing congestion and toxicity after surgery, an illness, or an emotionally and physically challenging time. Since these herbs can be depleting, do not take them continuously for longer than two weeks at a time.

Honor Nature's Rhythms

Nature functions in seasons, cycles, and rhythms. Every cell in our body has an intrinsic beat of rest and activity that evolved over millions of years of evolutionary time. Hormone levels, temperature regulation, immune function, digestive enzymes, sleep-wake cycles, and cellular reproduction all go through phases of rest and activity. In this age of technology we have the possibility of ignoring our internal biological clock and can stay up until two o'clock in the morning, eat our meals at any hour of the day or night, and sleep until noon. Despite our apparent freedom to disregard the rhythms of nature, our bodies pay a toll. Our lack of resonance with the environment contributes to insomnia, depression, concentration problems, and digestive ailments. Most of us have had the experience of jet lag, in which our inner clock is out of sync with the environment in which we arrive, and we feel disoriented and disconnected. By following a natural daily routine, we can improve the harmony between our inner and outer rhythms. Establishing an ideal daily routine is essential to enhancing our well-being. See if you can shift your choices in the direction of this recommended lifestyle pattern.

Herbs and Routine

No herb is going to force you into bed by ten o'clock, but a calming herb can help you drift off to sleep more effortlessly. A tea made from chamomile, valerian, hops,

Awaken around sunrise.
Empty your bowels and bladder.
Shower, brush your teeth, clean
    your tongue.
Meditate.
Eat breakfast if you are hungry.

Eat lunch at noon, preferably as
    your largest meal.
Take a walk after lunch.

Meditate before dinner.
Eat a light dinner, no later than
    seven o'clock.
Take a walk after dinner.

Have light evening activity.
Be in bed with the lights out no
    later than 10:30 P.M.

passionflower, or the Ayurvedic herb jatamansi can help quiet a turbulent mind and allow you to drift from waking into the sleeping state of consciousness. Even a cup of hot milk to which nutmeg, cardamom, or a few saffron threads are added can encourage restful sleep.

If you are having difficulty with regular daily elimination, several gentle herbal agents can help normalize digestion. Psyllium, flaxseed, or a classical Ayurvedic formula called Triphala are bulk-forming herbal products that enhance movement through the digestive tract without irritating the colon or creating bowel laziness. A diet rich in fresh fruits, vegetables, whole grains, and legumes will provide natural sources of the fiber that is essential to regular elimination.

If you have difficulty maintaining the energy level you need for success and joy in your life, first look at the basics of your daily routine, then consider adding a tonic herb to your diet. There is a class of Ayurvedic herbs known as *rasayanas* or rejuvenatives that provide a subtle level of nourishment. The primary woman's rasayana is a type of wild asparagus called shatavari. The primary men's rasayana comes from the root of the winter cherry bush, called ashwagandha in Sanskrit. Ginseng has an established tradition in Asia as a rejuvenative, and is receiving growing attention in the West. Other, more commonly known tonics include garlic, almonds, licorice, milk, and honey. Ingesting these nourishing substances can contribute to a healthy daily routine in which you have energy available when you need it.

Use Your Senses

We consume the world through our five senses. What we hear, touch, see, taste, and smell is metabolized into the chemistry and electricity of our body and can make the difference between health and sickness, life and death. Soothing, beautiful sounds can calm colicky babies, improve the immune response of a person with AIDS, and reduce the chance of surgical complications during an operation. Regularly immerse yourself in natural environments where the only sounds you hear are those of nature—the breeze rustling through the trees, the birds warbling in the bushes, the stream rushing over the rocks. These primordial sounds bring us back to our centered place of healing.

Stimulating our inner pharmacy through the sense of touch has been a feature of healing traditions around the world since the beginning of humanity. Using botanically derived, herbalized oils during massage can enliven the integration between mind and body. Sesame, almond, coconut, olive, sunflower, or jojoba oils to which sandalwood, jasmine flowers, neem, camphor, or ginger have been added can be soothing or enlivening, depending upon the plant added.

A daily self-massage is one of the simplest and most important therapeutic approaches we can do for ourselves. Try adding this ritual to your daily routine prior to your bath or shower, using a few tablespoons of a natural oil, warmed above body temperature.

Visual stimuli to which we are exposed also affect our well-being. Receiving uplifting rather than demoralizing visual input can trigger the release of our internal healing chemicals. Just looking at a bountiful, lush landscape can lower our blood pressure and reduce the level of circulating stress hormones. Spend time in your garden, hiking through the woods, or strolling in the park. Take in the sights of nature for their balancing and healing influence.

The fragrances of the world have a subtle yet profound effect on our mind and body. The surging interest in aromatherapy reflects our need to reconnect with nature. Essential oils derived from flowers, fruits, herbs, and spices enable us to take nature into our home environment. Almost any plant-based substance that can be ingested as an herb can be extracted to produce an essential oil. Lavender, rose, chamomile, nutmeg, and olibanum extracts are just a few of the many essential oils that can be used to calm and soothe. Juniper, ginger, cinnamon, rosemary, and cardamom are examples of aromatic oils that are stimulating and enlivening. Explore the fragrances derived from the plant kingdom and create an aromapharmacy for yourself.

Herbs and Wholeness

We are inextricably connected to the plant kingdom. The air we breathe and the food we eat, along with the sounds, sensations, sights, and smells that surround us, are

Performing an Oil Massage

Pour a tablespoon of warm oil on your scalp, massaging the oil in vigorously. Cover your entire scalp with small circular strokes, as if you were shampooing. Move to your face and ears, massaging more gently. Apply a little oil to your hands and massage your neck, front and back, then your shoulders.

Vigorously massage your arms, using a circular motion at the shoulders and elbows and long back-and-forth motions on the long parts. Using large, gentle, circular motions, massage your chest, stomach, and lower abdomen. A straight up-and-down motion is used over the breastbone. Apply a bit of oil to your hands and reach around without straining to massage your back and spine, using up-and-down motions.

Vigorously massage your legs as you did your arms, in a circular motion at the ankles and knees, straight back and forth on the long parts. With the remaining oil, vigorously massage your feet, with attention to the soles and toes.

Washing off the oil: Keeping a thin, almost undetectable film of oil on the body is considered beneficial for toning the skin and keeping the muscles warm during the day. Therefore, wash yourself with warm, not hot, water and mild soap.

infused with the essence of plants. We encourage you to consider your relationship with herbs as more than alternative medicines that you take for the inevitable uncomfortable symptoms of life. Rather, use your botanical friends to remind you about gaining and maintaining balance in life, through what you eat, the rhythms of your day, and your sensory experiences. We can use the herbal kingdom to point us in the direction of health, which, in essence, is a state of wholeness.

4   *Science-of-Life Herbology*

Drugs which
have been
observed to be
efficacious
from time
immemorial
should alone be
used in the
course of a
medical
treatment.
—SUSHRUTA
SAMHITA

The timeless wisdom of Ayurveda provides the framework for our healing programs at the Chopra Center for Well Being. The name itself expresses its all-encompassing domain. *Ayur* means "life" in Sanskrit, and *veda* means "knowledge." Ayurveda, then, is the knowledge or science of life. As an oral tradition passed down from generation to generation, Ayurveda has its roots in the mists of antiquity. As a codified body of wisdom, two major schools of Ayurvedic medicine are acknowledged. The Charaka school resembled our modern discipline of internal medicine, with a primary focus on the prevention and treatment of chronic disorders. Charaka strongly emphasized the importance of mind-body interactions in the promotion of health. The Sushruta school had a greater focus on the treatment of acute diseases, which included the development of many surgical procedures. Although there is ongoing debate concerning which sage lived earlier, most medical historians date Charaka and Sushruta to about the fourth or fifth century B.C. Considering how much we have learned about health and sickness over the past several millennia, it is remarkable how many of the ancient principles of Ayurveda remain relevant today.

According to Ayurveda, life is the harmonious interweaving of our environment, body, senses, mind, and spirit. Illness results when there is a loss of balance and integration between these layers. To establish and maintain good health, we need to understand our natural state of health and identify the tendencies that take us away from our optimal state of balance. One of the most important contributions of Ayurveda is the recognition that each of us metabolizes the energy and information of the environment in a unique way. The better we understand our intrinsic nature and how our environment influences our state of being, the better we can make choices to optimize our health.

Our inner and outer environments are organized according to five primary elements, described in Ayurveda as *space, air, fire, water,* and *earth.* Each of these principles represents a primary force that can be applied to the physical inanimate world, our living biology, and the workings of our mind. Let's explore these principles in more detail.

The first element, space, represents the potentiality principle from which all possible expressions of nature arise. Ultimately, the silent emptiness of space is the source of all the other elements. Although it is beyond the perception of the senses, space is the media in which all sensory experiences arise. In the language of modern physics, space is the unified field in which all the known forces of nature are expressed.

Space gives rise to the second element, air, which represents the movement principle that governs the motions of galaxies, the transport of biochemicals and the activity of subatomic particles. When the movement force flows smoothly within living systems, energy and information circulate freely, supporting healing and evolution.

The third element, fire, is the principle of transformation and metabolism. Nuclear reactions in stars are governed by this element, as is energy production in cells. This force regulates metabolism in the body and must be at an optimal level of functioning in order to accomplish its mission of energy production. As with a nuclear power plant or a fire in your fireplace, there is an ideal level of activity that allows the energy to be harnessed efficiently. Too much or too little fire can have harmful consequences.

The fourth element, water, represents the forces of attraction and cohesion. The gravitational pull between planets, the cohesive forces in a molecule, and the attraction of sweethearts in love are all manifestations of the water principle. Within biological systems, water is the stock of the living soup in which the chemistry of the body brews.

Finally, the earth principle is expressed as the matter of the physical universe. Modern physicists assure us that despite the appearance of solidity that our senses provide, all matter is ultimately nonmaterial, composed of condensed energy. Still, the planets, rocks, trees, bodies, organs, cells, and organelles that make up the stuff of everyday life do exist and are governed by the earth principle.

The Elements of Plants

The five primary forces come together in all life forms, where they are organized into cells, tissues, organs, and organisms. Health results from the harmonious interaction of all the forces and elements in our mind and body. Illness is a loss of this delicate equilibrium. When we experience an imbalance in our physiology, we can use the resources of our environment to reestablish harmony and balance.

Plants are elegant expressions of the primary elements, for all five forces are represented. They extract the elements from the earth and are our primary source of minerals and trace metals. Fortunately, plants have learned how to digest the earth so we don't have to eat dirt to get our daily helping of minerals. There are unique relationships between botany and geology, with certain plants having a special affinity for specific elements. Wild buckwheat likes to grow where there is an abundance of silver in the ground, wild poppy has an appetite for copper, and horsetail seems to prefer gold. The ability of plants to concentrate molecules of matter provides us with essential elements in forms that are digestible and absorbable. Certain herbs are inherently more grounding, carrying within them an abundance of the earth element. Examples of these heavier, denser herbs derived from roots include ashwagandha, marshmallow, shatavari, and lotus.

Plants have evolved elaborate systems to integrate the water element into their structure. From roots to leaves, from cacti to melons, water is an essential component of our botanical friends. Plants are abundant sources of moisture for animals, and are providers of many water-soluble healing chemicals. Although we consume an abundance of water when we eat fresh fruits and vegetables, most medicinal herbs are dried before we ingest them. Assuming this dehydration is performed with care, the extraction of water stops the metabolism of the plant but leaves the active chemicals to be released when we consume them. Medicinal herbs that are naturally rich in the water element include amalaki, aloe vera, slippery elm, and licorice.

The fire element is captured by plants through the process of photosynthesis, which converts solar energy into carbohydrates. When we consume plants and herbs, we liberate that energy for our benefit. Without this trapping of light by our botanical friends, we could not exist. Many herbs concentrate fire, an activity expressed in their pungency. Ginger, black pepper, cayenne, thyme, cloves, and cinnamon are fiery herbs that generate heat in the body when we consume them and can be used to kindle a weak digestive fire.

From an animal perspective, the air element is one of the prime reasons for the existence of plants. Plants are the lungs of our living planet, generating our oxygen and trapping our carbon dioxide waste gases. Many aromatic herbs, including the mints, fennel, camphor, cinnamon, rosemary, and jasmine, can be used therapeutically to improve respiratory function.

Certain herbs have unique effects on the nervous system that can be seen as expressing the element of space. These tend to be consciousness-altering or hallucinogenic substances that have the effect of temporarily expanding the mind. Because substances such as peyote, datura, marijuana, psilocybin, and ayuhausca are potentially dangerous and illegal in most countries, we won't be exploring them further in this book. Other, safer herbs that

influence the mind, such as *Gingko biloba* and gotu kola, will be explored.

The Elements of Humans

As creatures of the universe, we, too, are composed of the five primary elements. According to Ayurveda, the five primary forces can be reduced in human beings to three primary principles that govern our bodies and minds. The first principle, known as *Vata* in Sanskrit, is responsible for all movement within the physiology. Composed of a mixture of space and air, the motion principle regulates the movement of thought, muscles, circulation, digestion, and elimination. When the movement principle becomes aggravated or excessive, we experience anxiety, insomnia, tremor, palpitations, gaseousness, and constipation. We can settle the movement principle through grounding and calming behaviors, foods, and herbs.

The second mind-body principle, called *Pitta* in Sanskrit, is composed of the fire and water elements. Acting as a chemical fire, this principle is responsible for digestion and metabolism of matter or information we ingest from the environment. When the fire principle is aggravated, we experience heartburn, inflammation, skin rashes, hot flashes, and irritability. Herbs that have a cooling, soothing influence are useful in pacifying Pitta-aggravated conditions.

The third principle is *Kapha,* composed of the earth and water elements. Kapha is responsible for maintaining the structure and lubrication of our physiology. When it accumulates excessively, we experience retention and congestion. Sinus problems, weight gain, diabetes, excessive sleepiness, and fluid retention are manifestations of too much earth and water in the system. Herbs that have light, heating, and aromatic qualities are beneficial in the treatment of Kapha disorders.

According to the Ayurvedic framework, three issues need to be considered when approaching a health concern: the first is the nature of the illness, the second is the nature of the intervention, and the third is the nature of the person who has the health problem. Although in Western medicine once we diagnose a disease, we tend to treat it similarly in every person, this is not the case in many natural health care systems. As physicians, we may collectively label as migraines, headaches characterized by sharp pains that disturb sleep, those with burning pain that cause irritability, and those associated with a sense of congestion and nausea. From an Ayurvedic perspective, however, they reflect different imbalances and require different interventions.

Knowing the qualities of an herb is essential if we are to use it effectively. You don't want to take a depleting herb if your system is already run down, nor would you add predominantly pungent herbs to your diet if you were regularly overheating or having hot flashes. We'll discuss the useful defining characteristics of herbs a little later in this chapter.

Understanding the person who has the illness is as important as understanding the illness that has the person. People who naturally have more of one element in their nature will experience different manifestations of an imbalance or illness from someone who has a natural predominance of another element. They will also respond differently to treatment. Although medical doctors experience this phenomenon every day, we were not taught to ask, "Why did one patient have a good response to the medication, whereas another patient with similar symptoms had a very negative reaction?" Knowing more about a person's mind-body constitution can help personalize treatments.

If you have not identified the predominant mind-body principles in your nature, complete the following brief survey. Understanding the proportion of elements in your physiology can help you choose healing interventions that are most suited for you. For those who are interested, a more in-depth discussion of constitutional typing is available in our earlier books, *Perfect Health, The Wisdom of Healing,* and *Vital Energy.*

Mind-Body Principles

For each of the twelve traits listed below, see if you can identify one characteristic pattern that best applies to you. If you believe that two choices are equally applicable, you may circle both. Total your scores for each column to learn the relative proportion of the three principles in your nature.

Characteristic	Vata/ Motion "Wind"	Pitta/ Metabolism "Fire"	Kapha/ Structure "Earth"
ACTIVITY	active, restless	directed, precise	methodical, easy-going
UNDER STRESS	anxious	irritable	withdrawn
SLEEP	light, interrupted	short, but sound	deep and prolonged
APPETITE	variable	strong	steady
DIGESTION	irregular, gassy	sharp, acidic	slow
ELIMINATION	constipated, variable	loose, frequent	regular, formed
FRAME/ WEIGHT	light, thin	medium, average	broad, heavy
SKIN	dry	warm, moist	thick, soft
BODY TEMPERATURE	cold	warm	cool
TENDONS, VEINS	visible	moderate	hidden
ABDOMEN	thin	muscular	thick, soft
SPEECH	talkative	forceful	deep, resonant
Totals	Vata =	Pitta =	Kapha =

Interpreting Your Scores

Rank your tallies for Vata, Pitta, and Kapha from the highest to the lowest number. The highest score usually identifies the principle that is predominant in your mind-body nature. If the largest number is four or more points greater than the next principle, you can say that that principle is dominant in your physiology. For example, if your scores were Vata = 10, Pitta = 5 and Kapha = 3, Ayurveda would characterize your nature as having the greatest abundance of Vata, with less prominence of Pitta and Kapha. If your two highest scores are within three points of each other, then your inherent mind-body nature predominantly reflects the two top principles, with the third less represented. For example, if your scores were Vata = 4, Pitta = 8 and Kapha = 9, then you would be classified as Kapha/Pitta with Vata less prominent. Most people will have two principles within a few points of each other, with the third less represented. The rarest constitutional type is when all three principles are closely clustered. An example of this pattern would be Vata = 7, Pitta = 6 and Kapha = 5. People with this pattern are generally more tolerant of a wider range of foods, climates, and sensory experiences.

As you learn about the therapeutic effects of specific herbs, pay some attention to the influence they have on Vata, Pitta, and Kapha. If you have identified Pitta as the predominant energy in your nature, you may want to be cautious when ingesting an herb that has the tendency to aggravate Pitta. This additional level of understanding can be very helpful in effectively using herbal medicines.

Herbal Energetics

Herbs can influence mind and body in different ways. According to Ayurveda, the three primary levels that must be understood to maximize the value of an herbal medicine are (1) the proportion of elements as carried in the taste of the herb; (2) the heating or cooling potency of the herb; and (3) the special medicinal qualities that the herb possesses. As an example, nutmeg has a spicy, pungent taste. In Ayurvedic theory, the pungent taste is composed of the air and fire elements; therefore, taking nutmeg will add to the quantity of these elements in the system. It has a heating potency, and will therefore tend to increase the temperature and metabolic activity of the body. What we could not predict on the basis of its taste or potency is its sedative effect on the nervous system, which makes it an effective sleeping aid when taken in warm milk. Knowing its other qualities, however, you would use nutmeg more cautiously if you were feeling overheated or irritable.

Symptom-oriented herbology does not take into account the nature of the person or illness. The overall effect of echinacea may

Tastes and Elements	
Taste	Elements
sweet	earth and water
sour	earth and fire
salty	water and fire
pungent	fire and air
bitter	air and space
astringent	air and earth

not be beneficial in persons who have a predominance of Vata in their nature, particularly if their susceptibility to colds is triggered by poor nutrition and sleep/wake cycles. The use of ginger for morning sickness in a woman with high Pitta may increase her irritability. Before you take any herbal supplement, we recommend that you ask yourself the following questions:

1. What are the predominant qualities of the problem I am attempting to resolve? For example, if I have a lingering cough, is it dry or wet, scratchy or thick, cold or hot?

2. What are the predicted qualities of the herb, and what are its special qualities that may benefit my condition? For example, is the herb drying, moistening, purifying, or heating? Does it possess a specific anti-infectious quality that may help clear up a lingering bronchitis?

3. Knowing my predominant mind-body principles, are there any special precautions I should exercise? For example, if I am experiencing Vata aggravation, evidenced by anxiety, insomnia, and constipation, could this herb taken for my cough worsen my mental and physical turbulence?

Considering the greater context in which an herb is used honors its potency and enhances the prospect that the herb will have the desired effect on your well-being. Remember that herbs are gifts from nature and as such are deserving of our appreciation and respect. Ask from them what they are capable of providing and use them with discrimination. Keep in mind the wise words of Sushruta, one of the great Ayurvedic sages, who eloquently expressed the essence of effective medicines: "A medicine, too strong for the disease it has been applied to combat, not only checks it but may give rise to a fresh malady, because its surplus energy is not used up by the weakened and conquered distemper. . . . On the other hand, medicines of inadequate potencies, unequal to the strength of a disease, fail to produce any tangible effect. Therefore, only medicines of appropriate power should be administered."[1]

Appropriately applying the power of herbs allows us to tap into the healing power of nature. Great healers across time and space have understood that health is a state of dynamic balance and that nature is the supreme healer. The Upanishads describe our relationship to the elements and forces around us in this simple description of evolution:

"From consciousness arose space— from space, air—from air, fire—from fire, water—from water, earth—from earth, plants—from plants, food—from food, man."

Our botanical friends can help us regain and maintain the harmony we seek with nature and for this gift, we owe our deepest gratitude.

5

Restoring Balance, Creating Health

Rejoice plants,
bearing
abundant
flowers and
fruit,
triumphing
together over
disease like
victorious
horses,
sprouting forth,
bearing
humanity safe
beyond disease.
—RIG VEDA

According to Ayurveda, every illness progresses through stages of development before it becomes apparent. Even a simple cold does not spontaneously arise. The nasty viruses that cause the sneezing, congestion, and misery of an upper-respiratory infection incubate for days, hiding from and then overriding our immune defenses before filling our heads with phlegm. Other chronic diseases such as arthritis, heart disease, and cancer generally take years before they are fully entrenched and declare themselves with signs and symptoms.

Ayurveda describes the development of disease as moving through progressive stages of imbalance until the normal homeostatic mechanisms of our body are incapable of reestablishing equilibrium. If we accept this principle, the earlier we intervene therapeutically, the more likely we are to see a benefit. This is particularly true in the use of herbal medicines. Herbs can play an important role in helping to reestablish balance and are particularly effective if the illness has not fully manifested as abnormalities on blood tests or X-rays. The use of herbs in digestive disturbances, anxiety, insomnia, depression, fatigue, menstrual and menopausal discomforts, weight control, and chronic pain syndromes can be very rewarding. In these conditions, we think of herbal medicines as supplying a subtle form of nourishment to help replenish and restore physiological systems. When we recommend an herb for a patient with cancer, it is with the intention to reduce toxicity and strengthen immunity. If we suggest an herb for a woman going through menopause, it is to help restore balance during a time of physiological and emotional transition. Although herbs can effectively address specific symptoms and diseases, they are particularly helpful in strengthening the person with the problem, rather than solely as an attack on the problem itself. This approach derives from the model that disease is the absence of health, rather than health as the absence of disease. In this spirit let's explore various categories of illness and the role that herbs can play in reducing the distress and suffering that attend these problems.

Herbs for Digestion

Essential to health and well-being is our ability to digest packets of energy and information we derive from the environment and efficiently transform them into the energy and substance of our body. In Ayurveda, the body is known as *anna maya kosha,* which means the layer composed of food. Basically, our body is composed of molecules derived from food and directed by our DNA into the appropriate sites. Amino acids from the protein in the milk you had for breakfast may now be serving as a molecular girder in your biceps muscle. The sugar molecule carried in the tortilla you had for lunch may be providing energy to a nerve cell in your brain. The next time you consume a fruit salad, consider how the carbohydrates, proteins, fats, vitamins, minerals, and phytochemicals are being absorbed in your digestive tract and distributed to the cells and tissues throughout your body. When the processes of digestion, absorption, and elimination are occurring optimally, we take in the nutrition we require and eliminate the waste we don't need. Each stage of the nutritional process—the initial digestion of food in the mouth and stomach, the absorption of nutrients in the small intestines, and the elimination of waste from the colon—must be healthy for us to be healthy. And we can use herbs to enhance each phase of the digestive process.

STAGE 1. APPETITE AND DIGESTION

Appetite and digestion are closely linked and reflect the quality of our digestive fire, known as *agni* in Ayurveda. When our digestive fire is strong, we are able to break down the food we ingest into its basic elements, allowing for the appropriate sorting of components into those that are nourishing and those that are best eliminated. People can have problems with either too little or too much digestive fire, resulting in delicate digestion on the one hand and heartburn or acid indigestion on the other. Herbs to stimulate the digestive fire are generally spicy in nature and best taken immediately prior to or with a meal. Ginger, black pepper, cayenne, celery seeds, and long pepper contain essential oils that have effects at several levels of the digestive process. Studies from Germany, for example, have suggested that ginger stimulates the flow of salivary enzymes, activates stomach activity, and contains enzymes that help digest proteins.[1]

Bitter herbs can also enhance the first stage of digestion by way of a neural reflex between the tongue and our gastric stimulation center in the brain stem. The classical bitter digestive tonic is gentian, which enhances stomach emptying and stimulates the secretion of enzymes by the stomach, gallbladder, and pancreas. Other bitter herbs that are useful in small quantities to stimulate appetite and digestion include golden seal, aloe vera, and chamomile.

On the other end of the spectrum are those conditions in which there is excessive digestive fire. Hyperacidity, heartburn, gastroesophageal reflux, and peptic ulcers are expressions of an inefficient digestive fire that is imbalanced in both location and quantity. Cooling herbs that pacify the excessive heat and encourage a cleaner digestive fire can help reduce heartburn and improve digestion. These include cumin, coriander, fennel, and licorice as well as the Ayurvedic herbs amalaki and shatavari. They are generally taken after a meal or when the symptoms of acid indigestion are prominent.

STAGE 2. ABSORPTION AND TRANSIT

Once food leaves the stomach and enters into the intestines, our body is involved in the process of digesting and absorbing the essential nutrients required for meeting the energy and molecular needs of the body. Problems with this phase of digestion result in gas, bloating, and heaviness after a meal. People with assimilation difficulties often report that even though they are eating healthy foods, they do not feel they are being adequately nourished.

Herbs that assist with this phase help coordinate the movement of food through the intestines. Nutmeg, chamomile, peppermint, and lemon verbena are herbs traditionally used to reduce abdominal spasms and bloating. Cinnamon, cardamom, and bay are known as the "three carminatives" in Ayurveda, meaning that they help dispel congested intestinal gas. In people who are sensitive to dairy products but may not have an actual lactase deficiency, warming milk with cinnamon, cardamom, or nutmeg can often improve their tolerance. Other culinary herbs useful in reducing bloating include basil, oregano, thyme, coriander, cumin, dill, and fennel. Ayurvedic herbs useful in reducing gas that are not as well known in the West include wild celery seeds, nutgrass, and long pepper. If you are among the many people who experience bloating after eating beans or legumes, cooking with asafetida can improve digestive ability.

STAGE 3. ELIMINATION

Although we were taught in medical school that daily bowel movements were not required for good health, most people feel better if they are eliminating regularly. A fiber-rich diet, with plenty of fresh fruits, vegetables, and whole grains is the most important contributor to daily elimination. When necessary, adding fiber in the form of psyllium or flaxseed can invigorate sluggish bowels. A classic Ayurvedic formula called triphala consists of three fruits—amalaki, bibhitaki, and haritaki. Like psyllium, the fiber in triphala can help enhance elimination in people whose bowels are slow, and normalize bowel movements in people who tend toward loose stools.

Only rarely should an herbal stimulant cathartic be used. Castor oil, cascara sagrada, senna, and aloe are the most common plant-based laxatives that act by stimulating the nerve fibers to the colon and by causing the accumulation of salts and water in the intestines. These laxatives can cause abdominal cramping, with cascara the mildest and castor the strongest. The main problem with repeated use of these herbal stimulants is that the bowel gets lazier the more they are used. People who resort to them regularly often become trapped in a dependency cycle and cannot evacuate without the herbs. Usually, diet, exercise, and bulk-forming herbal remedies are sufficient to keep the bowels moving without resorting to stimulant cathartics. Good food is preferable to good medicines.

Herbs for the Mind and Emotions

Emotional ups and downs are a part of life. Many people go through periods when they are feeling enthusiastic and other times when the challenges of life feel overwhelming. Episodes of worry, anxiety, insomnia, and sadness affect people at all ages. Usually, with the passage of time, the wheel of life turns and uncomfortable emotions transform into more comfortable ones. But occasionally, distressing feelings persist, seeming to take on a life of their own, interfering with relationships and daily activities. When the emotional challenge is bothersome but not disabling, a trial of an herbal aid may provide needed support while the underlying life issue unfolds. In cases of mild anxiety, insomnia, and melancholy, herbs may provide sufficient relief to avoid the need for prescription medication. If you are in more severe emotional distress, however, we strongly encourage you to seek professional assistance and use all the resources of modern medicine available to get you through your difficult time.

Herbs that may be of value in supporting emotional balance can be classified into two categories, calming and enlivening. Calming herbs are beneficial when the mind is overly turbulent, generating worry and anxiety during the day and insomnia at night. Enlivening herbs can be helpful when fatigue and depression are clouding access to your inner source of energy. Modern science is just beginning to assess seriously the value of herbs to soothe and invigorate the mind and emotions.

CALMING HERBS

There is a long history of herbal approaches for soothing emotional turbulence. One of the best-known calming herbs is valerian root, used since the time of the Roman Empire. Studies have confirmed valerian's sedative properties, although its active components have yet to be conclusively identified. Hops, another valuable relaxing herb, has been prescribed to encourage sound sleep and pacify mental restlessness since the Middle Ages. A sachet of hops is traditionally placed under a child's pillow to deliver sleep-inducing aromatherapy. Another plant, passionflower has been shown to have calming activity in animals and is widely used in European herbal sedative formulas. Rapidly gaining in popularity as a natural sedative is kava kava, an important herb of the Pacific Islands, where it has been used in rituals and ceremonies for thousands of years. Studies have confirmed that kava possesses measurable anti-anxiety effects, possibly acting through mechanisms similar to the tranquilizing drug Valium.[2]

The Ayurvedic herbal pharmacy offers a number of herbs traditionally used to support emotional balance. Ayurveda distinguishes emotional distress according to which element is most imbalanced. If a person is having excessive mental turbulence with stressful, anxious thoughts, a Wind-pacifying herb such as jatamansi is favored. If irritability and anger are creating distress, cooling herbs such as brahmi or gotu kola are prescribed. When there is excessive accumulation of toxic, morbid emotions, purifying herbs such as sage or guggulu are recommended. Considering the subtler qualities of an emotional symptom can help fine-tune a therapeutic choice.

The Western herb St. John's wort is one of the most popular natural remedies in Europe for the treatment of depression and is currently receiving widespread interest in the United States as well. Several studies have attested to its efficacy in the treatment of mild to moderate depression.[3] Although it takes longer to act than most pharmaceutical antidepressant drugs, its safety profile makes it an attractive natural mood booster.

HERBS TO ENHANCE MENTAL PERFORMANCE

All of us would like to maintain optimal mental performance throughout our lifetime. Herbs purported to enhance mental function have been a part of the lore of healing traditions for thousands of years. Ginseng, gotu kola, brahmi, and ginkgo are among the best-known botanicals that have been promoted to improve memory and cognitive function. Traditional texts extol the virtues of these mind-enhancing herbs, although it has been challenging for science to convincingly document the benefits of many of these plants. The notable exception has been ginkgo, which has been the subject of several studies confirming its memory-improving potential in both animals and humans. Ginkgo is a potent antioxidant, but its demonstrated value in

slowing the progression of Alzheimer's disease almost certainly involves other mechanisms. An interesting recent animal study from Germany demonstrated that a combination of ginkgo and ginger could reduce anxiety without impairing memory, unlike pharmaceutical agents such as Valium, which characteristically sacrifice memory for their sedative effects.[4] It is obvious that there is a treasure chest of untapped herbs for the mind and emotions that are calling for scientific exploration. The next century may become the era of rediscovering nature's pharmacy.

Herbs to Enhance Women's Health

Women have traditionally used nature's botanical gifts during times of transition in their reproductive cycles—to relieve premenstrual distress, to provide support during pregnancy and labor, and to ease the symptoms of menopause. Often the same herbs are used throughout a woman's life and are classified as "female tonics." Black cohosh from America, chaste-tree berries from the Mediterranean region, and dong quai from China are the best-known herbs used to balance the female reproductive system. Although their precise mechanisms are not fully understood, there is scientific evidence that these traditional medicines work.

One of the most popular women's herbs is black cohosh, prized by Native

American woman for use during both reproductive and menopausal years. Studies have suggested that black cohosh can alleviate menopausal symptoms, although it is unclear exactly how it acts. Another popular botanical, vitex agnus-castus, comes from the berries of the chaste tree, once believed to inhibit sexual desire. Tinctures and tablets of this plant have traditionally been used to regulate menstrual periods as well as to relieve breast tenderness. In addition to its role in premenstrual symptoms, chaste tree is widely recommended to reduce uncomfortable symptoms in menopause, although scientific research in this realm is limited.

Although not as well known in the West, Ayurvedic herbs have a long history in support of a woman's physiology. Shatavari, or Indian asparagus, is the primary Ayurvedic female tonic used in India during both reproductive and post-menopausal years. There is some evidence that shatavari reduces uterine irritability, which may account for its reported benefit in premenstrual syndrome. From an energetic standpoint, most Ayurvedic women's herbs have cooling, soothing effects and are believed to pacify accumulated heat that causes the irritability of premenstrual syndrome (PMS) and the hot flashes associated with menopause. The juice of the aloe vera plant is another traditional Ayurvedic female tonic. Considered a cooling blood purifier, it is commonly used to alleviate the symptoms of PMS and menopause. Although there is considerable scientific research on its wound-healing value, aloe vera's impact on women's health has not yet been investigated by Western medicine.

In traditional Chinese medicine (TCM), dong quai has been used for thousands of years in the support of women's health, treating symptoms from menstrual cramping to menopausal hot flashes. Reports from China have highlighted the antioxidant and phytoestrogenic properties of dong quai, but a recent study from California failed to confirm a measurable estrogenic effect in menopausal women.[5] Further research will be necessary to see if scientific explanations for the traditional claims of women's tonics can be uncovered.

Herbs to Balance Metabolism

Obesity, with its many potential medical complications, is a serious problem in the Western world. More than one-third of Americans are overweight, a substantial increase from just ten years ago. It is natural that someone trying to lose weight would hope that a simple substance could make the process effortless. Unfortunately, this magical commodity has not yet been discovered. Balanced nutrition and regular physical activity remain the cornerstones of an effective weight-loss program.

Herbs with stimulant properties have been used to reduce the appetite and increase the metabolism. The Chinese herb ma huang, which contains the chemical ephedrine, can cause elevated blood pressure, rapid heart rate, and anxiety. When used in a carefully controlled fashion, ephedrine can be helpful in treating the symptoms of allergies and asthma, but the use of this chemical, either naturally or synthetically derived, is not warranted for weight loss. An Indian herb, *Garcinia cambogia,* the source of a chemical hydroxycitric acid, has been suggested to be an effective weight loss agent. However, the only placebo-controlled study to look at this herbal agent failed to confirm its efficacy.[6]

Since we are unlikely to discover an herb that magically suppresses the appetite or melts away fat, how can we use herbs in support of healthy metabolism? From an Ayurvedic perspective, weight gain represents a Kapha or Earth imbalance. Herbs that create lightness and heat help reduce excessive accumulation of body mass. In Ayurveda, there is a classical formula that includes three herbs to enhance the first phase of digestion, three to enhance tissue metabolism, three to foster elimination, and one to clear the blood.

Trikatu means "the three pungent spices." They have a heating effect on the system and enhance appetite and the digestive process. Although people with weight problems often perceive their appetite as a

Ayurvedic Metabolism Formula

Herbs to Enhance Digestion

TRIKATU
(black pepper, long pepper, dry ginger)

Herbs to Enhance Tissue Metabolism

TRIMADA
(chitrak, vidanga, musta)

Herbs to Foster Elimination

TRIPHALA
(amalaki, bibhitaki, haritaki)

Blood-Clearing Herb

guggulu

devouring enemy, being in tune with your appetite is the best way to ensure that you eat when you need to and stop when you don't. The three heating herbs that make up Trimada are not well known in the West and have not been rigorously researched. They share heating properties and are traditionally considered to help metabolize stored fat. Triphala has been discussed previously as a bowel tonic to encourage balanced elimination. Guggulu, derived from the resin of a plant that is a cousin to myrrh, has been shown to effectively lower cholesterol and triglyceride levels.

If you are trying to lose weight, our recommendation is to use herbs and spices to create meals that are delicious and balanced in the six tastes. This will ensure that you are not overeating because you are craving a taste, even though you have had enough food volume. Use herbs to kindle your digestive fire, enhance your metabolism, and encourage regular elimination. Practice conscious eating techniques and strive to fulfill your emotional needs with loving, nurturing relationships rather than with food. Herbs can be valuable allies in a weight-loss program, but cannot substitute for healthy eating, regular exercise, and love.

Herbs to Enhance Men's Health

Sexual potency and concerns about prostate gland function are the two major areas in which herbal medicines have been promoted for the benefit of men's health. Throughout the ages, men have sought a magic elixir to maintain or regain the potency of youth. In Ayurveda we have a category of herbs known as *vajikarana,* which are characterized in an understated manner as "producing a long lineage of progeny, providing quick sexual stimulation, enabling one to perform sexually with women uninterruptedly and vigorously like a horse, making one charming for women, promoting corpulence, and infallible and indestructible semen even in older persons, rendering one great, having a number of offspring like a sacred tree, branched profusely and commanding respect and popularity in society."[7]

Herbs such as amalaki and ashwagandha are reputed to provide these potent qualities. Like ginseng in China and Korea, these Ayurvedic herbs have powerful reputations that have thus far been difficult to characterize scientifically. Amalaki has potent antioxidant qualities, as does ashwagandha, but it is unclear how these properties influence male potency. Of interest is a recent Korean study of ginseng that suggests this ancient herb may work through a nitric oxide pathway, similar to the mechanism by which the recently fashionable Viagra works.[8] Studies are in progress around the world in attempts to characterize the efficacy and means of action of these traditional herbal medicines.

Yohimbine is a minor herbal medicine used to treat difficulties with erection. Derived from the bark of an African tree, *Pausinystalia yohimbe,* this chemical blocks the effects of nerves that constrict blood vessels. Although several studies have shown yohimbine to be mildly to moderately effective, it can cause anxiety, sweating, and nausea and should therefore be used with caution.

HERBS FOR THE PROSTATE

Enlargement of the prostate is one of the most common health concerns of men. By age fifty, almost half of all men will have microscopic evidence of benign prostatic hyperplasia (BPH) and by age eighty, almost 90 percent will show changes. A swollen prostate can cause difficulties with urination in many ways: it can make it difficult to start urinating, create problems with complete emptying, make it necessary to get up several times during the night, and predispose to bladder infections. Up to 25 percent of men may eventually require some form of surgery to help improve urinary flow. A number of new medicines are effective in treating the symptoms of BPH, but their side effects and expense are sometimes limiting. Herbal alternatives may play a cost-effective role in mild prostate enlargement, but every man should have an evaluation from a qualified physician before starting an herbal remedy to be certain that the symptoms are due to benign prostate enlargement and not prostate cancer.

The documented benefits of saw palmetto berry have transformed this Native American plant from a weed to a cash crop. A number of studies have confirmed its value in reducing the symptoms of prostate enlargement without serious side effects.[9] A lesser-known botanical medicine, *Pygeum africanum,* has also been shown to have measurable benefit on the symptoms of BPH, with improvement seen in both subjective and objective aspects of urination.

Ayurveda offers a number of substances to improve urinary flow in men. Purnanarva, gokshura, and shilajit each have a long history of usage, but none have been scientifically researched for the treatment of BPH. Studies on shilajit have demonstrated anti-inflammatory activity, but whether this has any impact on the prostate is uncertain. Used to alleviate painful urination, these substances have mild diuretic effects. In view of their long-established traditional usage, they deserve formal scientific study.

Herbs to Alleviate Pain, Arthritis, and Inflammation

As long as human beings have been in motion, they have experienced musculoskeletal aches and discomforts. Consequently, traditional healing systems around the world have sought and identified botanical substances to relieve pain. Our most potent narcotic pain relievers are derived from the juice of the poppy, a plant well known to the ancient Sumerians over five thousand years ago. The bark of the willow tree is the original source of salicylates, the basis of aspirin. Although a multitude of effective nonsteroidal anti-inflammatory medicines are available today, natural alternatives continue to gain in popularity.

Glucosamine and chondroitin sulfates are widely used in degenerative arthritis. Although they are not herbal products, they are mentioned here because they are currently among the most commonly used "natural" arthritis medicines. Controversy as to their efficacy abounds, but recent reviews have suggested that they do reduce pain and may slow or stabilize joint deterioration.[10]

Massaging the skin with herbalized oils has been used to reduce tissue pain for thousands of years. Oil from the wintergreen shrub, menthol from mint, camphor from the camphor tree, and capsaicin cream from chili peppers are rubbed over a sore joint or muscle to increase blood supply and reduce pain. Capsaicin, which depletes nerve endings of the neurotransmitter known as substance P, reduces the transmission of painful impulses. It has been useful in painful conditions ranging from diabetes to osteoarthritis.

Internally, many common herbs and spices have measurable anti-inflammatory effects, although their clinical relevance remains to be fully defined. Turmeric, basil, rosemary, thyme, and chamomile are a few of the many culinary herbs and spices that can cool inflammation.

Frankincense and myrrh, gifts of the Three Wise Men to the Christ Child, are closely related to two Ayurvedic herbs used in the treatment of arthritis. An extract of *Boswellia serrata,* a close cousin to frankincense, has shown anti-inflammatory activity in both animals and people. Guggulu, the resin from *Commiphora mukul,* is in the same family as myrrh *(Commiphora molmol).* A number of recent studies attest to the long-standing reputation of guggulu as an effective anti-inflammatory agent.[11]

Finally, feverfew, an herb used for over two thousand years to treat headaches, is effective in the treatment of migraines and arthritis. Phytochemicals in this daisylike plant inhibit inflammation and muscle spasm. New users of feverfew should be cautious, as allergic reactions to this herbal medicine are not rare.

Herbs can be helpful in reducing the discomfort of chronic discomforts, but it is important to remember that pain is a symptom of some underlying dysfunction or imbalance. If a part of your body continues to call for attention, please have a competent health-care provider evaluate your symptoms to be certain that you are not ignoring an underlying illness that requires more-specific treatment.

Herbs to Enhance Immunity

Like animals, plants face challenges from their environment. Bacteria, viruses, and fungi seek the energy and nutrition that plants capture, just as animals do, and plants have evolved sophisticated defense mechanisms to protect themselves from hostile creatures. We may gain some immunologic advantage by eating certain herbs, perhaps because the same chemicals that protect the plants from microorganisms may support our immune system. Many Native American, Ayurvedic, and Chinese herbal medicines have been used traditionally to strengthen immunity. Laboratory and animal studies have confirmed that many plants have an influence on the immune system. Research documenting the value of these botanical medicines in humans is relatively scarce, but suggestive of measurable benefit.

The most popular immune-enhancing herb in the West is echinacea. Although it is not directly toxic to germs, echinacea does enhance several aspects of the immune system. Native to North America, both the flowers and roots of this purple coneflower have therapeutic value ranging from treating the common cold to healing wounds. Echinacea is often combined with another Native American herb, goldenseal. Although there has not been any convincing support of goldenseal as having immune-enhancing effects, it contains a chemical called berberine that has antibacterial activity.

The Chinese herb astragalus has been used for thousands of years to enhance resistance to infection. Studies over the past several years have confirmed its ability to enliven components of the immune system.[12] The most effective way to use both echinacea and astragalus is uncertain. Although some herbalists recommend taking echinacea throughout the cold and flu season, there is some evidence to suggest that its potency wanes after a couple of weeks. Therefore it should probably be taken at the first sign of a viral illness and continued for a week to ten days.

Ayurveda has its own offering of herbs that enliven immunity. Ashwagandha is among the most popular Ayurvedic herbs that have been shown to influence the immune system. In several studies, it seems to reduce the toxic effect of cancer chemotherapy drugs on the bone marrow. At least part of its effect is probably due to its antioxidant activity.

Another little-known Ayurvedic herb that has shown promising immune-enhancing properties is guduchi, also known as *amrit* (Sanskrit for immortality). This herb has demonstrated the ability to stimulate both antibody production and cellular immunity in animals.[13] Amalaki and shatavari are other Indian herbs traditionally used to nourish the subtle substance of immunity known as *ojas*. According to Ayurveda, when ojas is abundant and circulating, cells and tissues function optimally and in support of the whole physiology. Depletion of ojas makes us vulnerable to internal and external challenges. As with most Ayurvedic herbs, there has been little formal scientific research to date on these revered plants, but interest is growing to explore their possible clinical benefits.

Herbs for Detoxification

Other than poisoning by industrial or environmental toxins, the concept of toxicity is generally rejected by Western medicine, while the idea that we store toxins in our body that can interfere with normal physiological functions is a common principle of natural healing systems. From an Ayurvedic perspective, accumulated toxins, known as *ama,* result from poor eating habits, exposure to alcohol and drugs, and environmental pollutants. Imbalancing life stresses can also result in toxic accumulations, manifesting as fatigue, weakened appetite, and susceptibility to infection. Many people today who are labeled with the diagnosis of chronic fatigue or systemic candidiasis are considered by Ayurveda to have ama accumulations.

Perhaps a bridge between the long-standing natural healing systems and modern medical science is the recognition that free radical molecules can damage healthy tissues, leading to an accumulation of chemicals that interfere with normal cellular function. Smoking, high-fat diets, environmental toxins, radiation, and potent chemi-cals can increase the production of free radicals, accelerating the development of illnesses ranging from Alzheimer's disease to cancer, from arthritis to heart disease.

Many of the herbs traditionally used to detoxify the body contain antioxidant components and phytochemicals that help the body neutralize damaging free radical molecules. Allspice, clove, oregano, pepper, rosemary, sage, and turmeric have all been shown to possess potent antioxidant abilities. Herbs and spices were used in ancient times to reduce food spoilage. Today we are learning that they help protect our cells from damaging reactive molecules.

Among the most important detoxifying Ayurvedic herbs is ginger. One of its Sanskrit names is *vishwabhesaj,* which is translated as "universal medicine." From an Ayurvedic perspective, ginger enhances all phases of digestion and helps to reduce the accumulation of ama. From a scientific viewpoint, ginger has antioxidant properties and can reduce nausea and enhance digestive enzymes. Another important Ayurvedic detoxifier is aloe vera juice. It also is rich in antioxidants and is useful for a variety of chronic disorders including inflammatory conditions and liver problems.

A lesser-known detoxifying herb is neem, traditionally used to treat fevers and inflammation. It can enhance immunity and is highly regarded in India for its antiseptic and purifying properties. Neem is protective against yeast and bacterial infections and has been used in the treatment of malaria. It can induce abortions and should not be used by pregnant women.

Several herbs have been gaining attention for their possible protective role in conditions of liver damage. Kutki, phyllanthus, and silybum are traditional botanical medicines that have been shown to reduce liver damage as a result of injury by drug or infection.[14] From a natural medicine perspective, they support the liver in its detoxifying role.

Herbs for Rejuvenation and Energy

Herbal tonics and elixirs have been components of healing systems around the world for thousands of years. As people grow older, it is understandable that they seek out substances that promise to restore vitality and slow the aging process. Of course, if such a magic potion were reliable, we would have it in our water supply and there would be scant need for cosmetic surgeons.

As we discussed earlier, there is a growing recognition of the role of free radicals in the aging process. Biological molecules damaged by these reactive substances accumulate in cells and eventually interfere with normal functioning. Enhancing our ability to neutralize free radicals before they wreak their havoc is the basis of new treatments for several degenerative conditions including Parkinson's disease, Alzheimer's, heart disease, and multiple sclerosis.

We may learn that traditional herbal "tonics" provide value through their special chemical properties. The fruit of amalaki is one botanical substance that may deserve its reputation as a rejuvenative. It has been shown to be one of the richest sources of vitamin C available on earth. Studies in animals of formulas containing amalaki have suggested that it may confer protection against both heart disease and cancer.[15]

Ashwagandha, from the Ayurvedic tradition, and ginseng, from the traditional Chinese and Korean medical systems, are two herbs that play similar roles. Both are reputed to enhance energy and vitality, and are important rejuvenatives. The lore about these substances goes further, promising the recovery of the potency of youth. Is there a way to assess scientifically the claims of these almost mythical substances?

If we look at the idea of a rejuvenative from a modern perspective, what would we want it to accomplish? Simply speaking, we would like the herb to neutralize the damaging and degenerative effects of stress on mind and body. The Russians coined the term *adaptogen* to describe this protective effect. When animals are subjected to threatening situations, they respond with rises in stress hormones and weakness in the immune system. An adaptogen blunts the response of harmful effects of stress, and both ginseng and ashwagandha have shown some effectiveness in this regard. Whether this blunting of the stress response is due to antioxidant properties or some other effects is still to be defined. What is clear is that these tonic herbs have been around a long time and are likely to grow in popularity as our society ages.

In addition to tonic herbs, both traditional Chinese medicine (TCM) and Ayurveda emphasize the tonic value of specific foods. In TCM, rice, walnuts, and grapes are considered to be rejuvenating. In Ayurveda, milk, honey, almonds, and clarified butter are viewed as having specific tonic properties. In both Ayurveda and TCM, tonic foods are not recommended until after one has undergone a detoxification program. As more westerners embrace these principles, it will be interesting to see how we are able to integrate the concepts of detoxification and purification with our Western molecular medical model. If scientists take these ideas seriously enough to approach them with an open mind, we are certain that new discoveries of the healing value of natural substances will unfold.

Herbs to Enhance Circulation

Although the modern description of the circulatory system is generally credited to William Harvey in 1628, an understanding of the channels of circulation carrying energy and vital fluids to the tissues of the body was known to ancient Chinese and Indian physicians. Ancient healers also recognized that blockages to circulatory flow resulted in illness and death. Herbal medicines to improve circulation have been explored around the world, and many of them have been essential in the development of modern medicines. Digitalis, the heart stimulant, is derived from foxglove, an important cardiac tonic prized by the ancient Egyptians, and the blood pressure medicine called reserpine is an extract of snakeroot, well known to Ayurvedic doctors since antiquity. Because of the wide natural variation in the potency of these botanical medicines, the standardization of pharmacologically derived drugs was a major advance in the safe use of these powerful substances.

Circulatory herbs that are less potent and less risky can be grouped into three main categories: those that reduce fats in the blood, those that have a thinning effect on the blood, and those that have a tonic effect on the heart. Garlic and guggulu fall into the first category. Although many earlier reports suggested that garlic had a modest fat-lowering effect, a recent study has cast some doubts on this property.[16] Guggulu, the resin from a small native Indian tree, has consistently shown itself as a safe and effective lipid-lowering herb.

The tendency for blood to stagnate or clot contributes to the risk of cardiovascular attacks. Low daily doses of aspirin have been shown to reduce the risk of heart attacks and strokes. A variety of herbs and spices have been shown to affect platelets, the tiny blood components that initiate the clotting process. Turmeric, cumin, feverfew, and onions all keep platelets from sticking together too easily, although their clinical effectiveness remains to be defined. Although garlic's role in lowering blood lipids may be controversial, its effect on platelets is generally well accepted.

Circulatory tonics have a supportive effect on the heart. In the West, hawthorn has been used since the Middle Ages. It increases blood supply to the heart, inhibits the development of atherosclerosis, strengthens heart contractions, and mildly lowers blood pressure. These combined effects improve the quality of life in people with heart disease.[17] The Ayurvedic equivalent of hawthorn is arjuna, the bark of a tree that has been used in India for over three thousand years. Studies have suggested that this ancient heart tonic can reduce cholesterol levels, improve the strength of heart

contractions, and lower the frequency of chest pain episodes.[18] Although these herbal heart tonics may offer new approaches to the treatment of our society's most common serious illness, we strongly recommend that you consult with your physician before using them.

Honor Herbs and Be Smart

Herbs are nature's gifts. Used appropriately and respectfully, they can serve as valuable tools on the path toward regaining and maintaining your health. As with any tool, a medicinal herb can be useful in some circumstances, but not in all. Learning to use plant-based medicines in the right context and with the right intention is vital to tapping into their healing power.

If you are facing a serious illness, engage your physician in an open discussion of your needs. If you do not feel you can honestly explore your interest in natural healing approaches with your doctor, seek out a health-care provider who supports your role as an active partner in your healing journey. If you are taking medication for a problem, do not abruptly discontinue it without the guidance of your doctor. If you are on medication and wish to start an herbal remedy, discuss it with your health-care provider to be certain that there are not potentially dangerous interactions between the medicine and the herb.[19]

Used responsibly, plant-based medicines are important and valuable healing aids, but they are neither a substitute for necessary medication nor good nutrition. If we are to see the return of herbal medicines to their rightful place in our modern healing inventory, we need to use them judiciously. It is in this spirit of honoring the rightful place of herbs that we explore in detail the forty herbs that constitute the Chopra Center Herbal Formulary in the next section of this book. Most common health concerns can be addressed with these few dozen healing plants. We encourage you to become intimately familiar with them, as they can be your powerful healing allies.

6 Making the Best Use of This Book

The next major section is the heart of this book, in which we describe in detail the forty most important herbs in use at the Chopra Center for Well Being. In each description the familiar, Latin, and Sanskrit (when available) names are provided for each herb. After a brief introduction to the herb, we review the scientific research that has been published on the plant or its derived components. We share with many of our readers an aversion to unnecessary animal testing; still, we have chosen to reference all published sources that provide credible information that can help us advance the cause of natural choices in health care. To the spirits of the creatures that have been sacrificed in the name of science, we offer our deepest gratitude.

Following the scientific review is a description of the practical uses of the herb, which draws upon both ancient and modern healing systems. The traditional uses of an herbal product may be different from the popular applications, which are often based upon scientific findings. We feel most confident when there is alignment between the traditional and scientifically supported uses.

Next, we address the currently available forms of the herbal medicine in the marketplace, including usual dosing recommendations. Several studies have found that not every herbal product delivers on what it is advertised to be. In lieu of regulations and enforcement of herbal product quality, you must take the responsibility for ensuring that you are receiving high-quality herbs. Research the manufacturer, and favor those lines that produce a standardized product. A list of the constituents in our Chopra Center Herbal Formulary product line is provided in the appendix.

Each herb is then analyzed from an Ayurvedic perspective. Two-thirds of the herbs we explore in detail are traditional Ayurvedic medicines, with the remainder representing botanical substances derived from Native American, European, Chinese, and Australian herbal systems. Even if the herb was not originally known in India, we analyze it according to basic Ayurvedic principles, which elaborate its effects on the primary mind-body elements.

Finally, we address any potentially negative effects related to use of the herb. Precautions or known adverse side effects are reviewed. As a general principle, we do not encourage the use of herbal medicines in conjunction with pharmaceutical drugs unless you are under the guidance of a health-care provider who can help you navigate safely in both worlds. Similarly, because so little research has been done in this area, we recommend that you do not take medicinal herbs while pregnant or nursing a baby.

At the end of each description is a table that includes the ten basic physiological systems that may be influenced by the herb under discussion.

On pages 56–57 is a chart that covers each of the forty herbs, listed in alphabetical order according to their Latin names and showing their primary uses. A table of the alphabetized Latin, common, and Sanskrit names is presented on pages 58 to 61.

We hope this deeper exploration of herbal medicines will serve both individuals in their personal path to well-being as well as members of the professional health-care community. The botanical kingdom has provided us with vast natural healing resources, for which we are inexhaustibly grateful. We are in complete accordance with Linnaeus, the great eighteenth-century Swedish botanist when he wrote:

"Herbs and plants are medical jewels gracing the woods, fields, and lanes, which few eyes see, and few minds understand. Through this want of observation and knowledge, the world suffers immense loss."

THE
FORTY HERBS
OF THE
CHOPRA CENTER
HERBAL
FORMULARY

The Forty Herbs of the Chopra Formulary

	Circulatory/ Respiratory	Detoxifier	Digestive	Immune Enhancer	Men's Health	Metabolic	Nervine	Rejuvenative	Rheumatic	Women's Health
Allium sativum	X		X			X		X	X	
Aloe vera		X	X							X
Andrographis paniculata	X	X	X	X						
Asparagus racemosus			X	X				X		X
Astragalus membraneceus	X			X				X		
Azadirachta indica		X		X		X			X	
Boswellia serrata	X		X						X	
Camellia sinensis	X			X		X				
Cassia augustifolia		X	X							
Centella asiatica		X					X	X		
Cimicifuga racemosa									X	X
Coleus forskohlii	X									
Commiphora mukul	X	X				X			X	
Crataegus oxyacantha	X									
Curcuma longa		X	X						X	
Echinacea purpurea		X		X						
Eletteria cardamomum	X		X				X	X		
Emblica officinalis	X		X	X	X			X	X	
Ginkgo biloba	X						X			X
Glycyrrhiza glabra	X		X	X					X	

The Forty Herbs of the Chopra Formulary

	Circulatory/ Respiratory	Detoxifier	Digestive	Immune Enhancer	Men's Health	Metabolic	Nervine	Rejuve- native	Rheumatic	Women's Health
Gymnema sylvestre						X				
Hypericum perforatum							X			
Lavandula angustifolia			X				X			X
Linum usitatissimum	X		X						X	
Melaleuca alternifolia		X								X
Mucuna pruriens					X		X	X		
Ocimum sanctum	X		X	X		X				
Phyllanthus niruri	X									
Picrorhiza kurroa	X	X	X							
Piper methysticum							X			
Serenoa repens					X					
Silybum marianum		X								
Tanacetum parthenium							X		X?	
Terminalia arjuna	X	X	X							
Tinospora cordifolia		X		X				X		
Trigonella foenum-graecum	X		X			X		X		
Ulmus rubra	X		X					X		
Valeriana officinalis							X			
Withania somnifera				X	X		X	X		
Zingiber officinale	X	X	X				X	X	X	

Herbs Alphabetized According to Their Latin Names

	LATIN NAME	COMMON NAME	SANSKRIT NAME
1.	*Allium sativum*	garlic	rasonam
2.	*Aloe vera*	aloe	kumari
3.	*Andrographis paniculata*	Indian gentian	kirata, kalmegha, bhunimb
4.	*Asparagus racemosus*	wild asparagus	shatavari
5.	*Astragalus membraneceus*	astragalus	—
6.	*Azadirachta indica*	Persian lilac, neem	nimba, arishta
7.	*Boswellia serrata*	Boswellin	shallaki, kunduru
8.	*Camellia sinensis*	tea	chai
9.	*Cassia angustifolia*	senna	rajavriksha, markandika
10.	*Centella asiatica*	gotu kola	brahmi
11.	*Cimicifuga racemosa*	black cohosh	—
12.	*Coleus forskohlii*	coleus	pashanbhedi, balaka
13.	*Commiphora mukul*	gum gugal	guggulu
14.	*Crataegus oxyacantha*	hawthorn	—
15.	*Curcuma longa*	turmeric	haridra
16.	*Echinacea purpurea*	echinacea	—
17.	*Eletteria cardamomum*	cardamom	ela
18.	*Emblica officinalis*	Indian gooseberry	amalaki
19.	*Ginkgo biloba*	ginkgo	—
20.	*Glycyrrhiza glabra*	licorice	yasthimadhu

Herbs Alphabetized According to Their Latin Names

	LATIN NAME	COMMON NAME	SANSKRIT NAME
21.	*Gymnema syvlestre*	gurmar	mehasringi
22.	*Hypericum perforatum*	St. John's wort	—
23.	*Lavandula angustifolia*	lavender	—
24.	*Linum usitatissimum*	flaxseed	uma
25.	*Melaleuca alternifolia*	tea tree	—
26.	*Mucuna pruriens*	cowage plant	atmagupta, kapikacchu
27.	*Ocimum sanctum*	holy basil	tulsi
28.	*Phyllanthus niruri*	phyllanthus	bhymyaamlaki, bahupatra
29.	*Picrorhiza kurroa*	picroliv	kutki
30.	*Piper methysticum*	kava kava	—
31.	*Serenoa repens*	saw palmetto	—
32.	*Silybum marianum*	milk thistle	—
33.	*Tanacetum parthenium*	feverfew	—
34.	*Terminalia arjuna*	arjuna myrobalan	arjuna
35.	*Tinospora cordifolia*	amrit	guduchi
36.	*Trigonella foenum-graecum*	fenugreek	medhika, methi
37.	*Ulmus rubra*	slippery elm	—
38.	*Valeriana officinalis*	valerian	tagara
39.	*Withania somnifera*	winter cherry	ashwagandha
40.	*Zingiber officinale*	ginger	andraka, sunthi

Herbs Alphabetized According to Their Familiar Names

COMMON NAME	LATIN NAME	SANSKRIT
aloe	*Aloe vera*	kumari
amrit	*Tinospora cordifolia*	guduchi
arjuna	*Terminalia arjuna*	arjuna
astragalus	*Astragalus membraneceus*	—
black cohosh	*Cimicifuga racemosa*	—
boswellin	*Boswellia serrata*	shallaki, kunduru
cardamom	*Eletteria cardamomum*	ela
coleus	*Coleus forskohlii*	pashanbhedi, balaka
cowage plant	*Mucuna pruriens*	atmagupta, kapikacchu
echinacea	*Echinacea purpurea*	—
fenugreek	*Trigonella foenum-graecum*	medhika, methi
feverfew	*Tanacetum parthenium*	—
flaxseed	*Linum usitatissimum*	uma
garlic	*Allium sativum*	rasonam
ginger	*Zingiber officinale*	andraka, sunthi
ginkgo	*Ginkgo biloba*	—
gotu kola	*Centella asiatica*	brahmi
gum gugal	*Commiphora mukul*	guggulu
gurmar	*Gymnema sylvestre*	mehasringi
hawthorn	*Crataegus oxyacantha*	—

Herbs Alphabetized According to Their Familiar Names

COMMON NAME	LATIN NAME	SANSKRIT
holy basil	*Ocimum sanctum*	tulsi
Indian gentian	*Andrographis paniculata*	kirata, kalmegha, bhunimb
Indian gooseberry	*Emblica officinalis*	amalaki
kava kava	*Piper methysticum*	—
lavender	*Lavandula angustifolia*	—
licorice	*Glycyrrhiza glabra*	yasthimadhu
milk thistle	*Silybum marianum*	—
Persian lilac, neem	*Azadirachta indica*	nimba, arishta
phyllanthus	*Phyllanthus niruri*	bhymyaamlaki, bahupatra
picroliv	*Picrorhiza kurroa*	kutki
saw palmetto	*Serenoa repens*	—
senna	*Cassia angustifolia*	rajavriksha, markandika
slippery elm	*Ulmus rubra*	—
St. John's wort	*Hypericum perforatum*	—
tea	*Camellia sinensis*	chai
tea tree	*Melaleuca alternifolia*	—
turmeric	*Curcuma longa*	haridra
valerian	*Valeriana officinalis*	tagara
wild asparagus	*Asparagus racemosus*	shatavari
winter cherry	*Withania somnifera*	ashwagandha

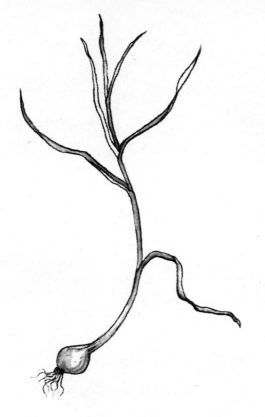

ALLIUM
SATIVUM

FAMILIAR: **garlic**
LATIN: *Allium sativum*
SANSKRIT: rasonam

Garlic declares its presence with its unmistakable pungent aroma. Its penetrating fragrance heralds its potent medicinal qualities, which have been identified and prized around the world. In Ayurveda it is considered a rejuvenative that nourishes all the tissue layers.

A native to central Asia, garlic was well known to the ancient Chinese, Greeks, Romans, and Egyptians. The slaves who built the Great Pyramid were fed garlic to improve their endurance.

In 1858, Louis Pasteur, the great French scientist who developed the process of pasteurizing milk, was the first westerner to document garlic's anti-infective properties, known to herbalists for thousands of years. Its has a long-standing reputation as a healing ally in cardiovascular disease and cancer. Thousands of scientific studies have been published on this complex botanical substance that contains almost two hundred different chemical components, most of which have not been carefully researched. Other than its strong odor, which unabashedly announces the presence of its aficionados, garlic has a very high safety profile as both food and medicine.

BOTANICAL AND PHYTOCHEMICAL INFORMATION

The characteristic fragrance of garlic is not released until the clove is broken and the odorless substance alliin makes contact with the enzyme allinase to create the familiar-smelling compound allicin. Allicin is not a stable compound and is further broken down by stomach acid and heat into a number of other sulfur-containing chemicals. Although most medical research has focused on allicin, these other components of garlic may also play important health-promoting roles. In addition to its chemical constituents, garlic is a good source of vitamins and trace minerals, including selenium. Although garlic has the greater reputation as a healing herb, onions also have similar sulfur-containing substances that may provide comparable benefits.

THE SCIENCE OF GARLIC

Garlic has been promoted as a natural protector against heart disease. Its potential benefits derive from its effects on blood lipids, clotting factors, and blood pressure. Several reports in the mid-nineties suggested that garlic was capable of lowering cholesterol levels by about 10 percent.[1, 2] More closely controlled subsequent studies produced inconsistent results, with some demonstrating definite benefit while others showed no value.[3, 4] For example, a recent report in the *Journal of the American Medical Association* did not find any lowering of high cholesterol levels in people who took steam-distilled garlic oil.[5] One of the challenges in making sense of these contradictory findings is that different forms of garlic are used in each study. In some reports, less than 10 percent of commercial garlic preparations contain even measurable allicin levels. Until we know what forms of garlic are most effective, we recommend you simply add garlic to your diet and enjoy the flavor, knowing that it may also be helping to lower your cholesterol level.

Garlic has other potential benefits on the cardiovascular system other than its possible role on fats in the blood. It inhibits the stickiness of platelets, reducing the tendency for blood vessels to clot.[6] Garlic also seems to keep blood vessels from becoming stiff, which may explain its ability to lower blood pressure.[7, 8] Although each property of garlic needs further documentation, its combined effects support the addition of this rich and complex herb to the diet of anyone who is concerned about heart disease.

Does the deodorized form provide equivalent benefits? Thus far, it is not clear what, if anything, is lost when the powerful-smelling allicin is neutralized. Enteric-coated forms may diminish the smell of garlic on your breath and skin without losing the therapeutic benefits.

Garlic's role in the prevention and treatment of cancer has received considerable attention. Studies in animals have shown that garlic reduces the risk of chemically caused tumors and can treat certain types of cancer in doses that are proportionate to what humans can get in their diet.[9, 10] Garlic added to human colon cancer cells grown in a laboratory is also effective in inhibiting their growth.[11]

Studies in people have shown that a diet rich in garlic may provide protection against stomach and breast cancer, although further research is needed to see how meaningful this effect is.[12, 13]

Garlic's role as an anti-infective agent is receiving renewed interest. It has been known for years to diminish the growth of viruses, bacteria, and fungi. Recent studies have suggested that garlic oil may help treat disease-producing agents ranging from athletes foot to *Pneumocystis carinii,* a serious infection commonly seen in AIDS patients.[14, 15] One of the most practical therapeutic applications of garlic may be its role in the treatment of *Helicobacter pylori,* a bacteria that has been associated with stomach ulcers and stomach cancer.[16] The usual treatment for this infection involves several expensive medications. If further studies confirm its efficacy, garlic may be a cost-effective treatment for this common condition.

THE PRACTICAL USE OF GARLIC

The repertoire of illnesses to which garlic has traditionally been applied is vast. Garlic has a reputation as an effective treatment for lung congestion, arthritic stiffness and pain, and to calm people with hysteria. It has been used to promote normal menstruation in woman and to improve libido in men. Applied externally, garlic oil is used as a liniment for sore muscles and to hasten the healing of festering sores. In addition to its role in heart disease and cancer, garlic is a natural pharmacy unto itself that can keep medical scientists busy for many years researching its potential therapeutic uses.

We use garlic as a grounding rejuvenative for people who have a predominance of mental turbulence. For those with mildly elevated cholesterol or high blood pressure, a daily clove of garlic added to sautéed vegetables or pasta sauce may reduce the need for medication. For people with recurrent peptic ulcers, it may be worth a trial of a couple of cloves of garlic per day before starting the prolonged antibiotic therapy that is usually required to eliminate the infectious agent associated with ulcers. For stubborn skin infections, apply freshly squeezed garlic oil directly to the area three times a day for a week. For people who cannot tolerate the strong smell of garlic or wish to avoid it for other reasons, leeks can provide similar but less odoriferous benefits.

HOW TO USE GARLIC

Garlic is available in many different forms, including capsules, tablets, and powders. It can be deodorized or enteric-coated. Although the precise chemicals and dosage that deliver garlic's benefits are still being defined, a daily clove of raw garlic is probably your safest bet that you are consuming adequate quantities of allicin. If you are taking a processed garlic product, try to find one that delivers a daily allicin dose of 4 to 5 milligrams (4,000 to 5,000 micrograms).

AYURVEDA AND GARLIC

Ayurveda has long recognized the healing potency of garlic, which carries five of the six tastes, missing only sour. It is balancing to Vata and Kapha, but has a moderately heating influence that may aggravate Pitta. You may read in Ayurvedic books that garlic is to be used sparingly by those engaged in spiritual practices because it has a dulling effect on the mind. Others suggest that it stimulates sexual passion and therefore is distracting for those on a spiritual path. If you are a monk or a nun, you may want to reduce your garlic use. For anyone else, a little garlic may help enhance your health and well-being.

PRECAUTIONS

Precautions with garlic follow its therapeutic effects. If you are on blood-pressure medications and begin taking regular doses of garlic, be certain to monitor your pressures so you are not overtreating your hypertension. Because of garlic's potential blood-thinning properties, be cautious taking garlic if you are on blood-thinning medicines.

Circulatory/Respiratory	Detoxifier	Digestive	Immune Enhancer	Men's Health
X		X		
Metabolic	Nervine	Rejuvenative	Rheumatic	Women's Health
X		X	X	

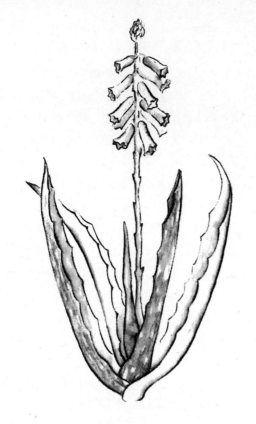

ALOE
VERA

FAMILIAR: **aloe vera**
LATIN: *Aloe vera*
SANSKRIT: kumari

Aloe vera has been honored as a healing plant for thousands of years around the world. The ancient Mesopotamians, Egyptians, and Greeks knew of the therapeutic benefit of this hardy succulent. In Ayurveda, aloe is known as *kumari,* which, alluding to its recuperative properties, can be translated as "the vitality of youth." There are several hundred species of aloe plants, of which aloe vera is best known for its medicinal qualities. Native to southern and eastern Africa, aloe is now cultivated throughout the Mediterranean, India, the Caribbean, and Australia. Thriving easily as an indoor potted plant, families on almost every continent keep aloe close at hand to treat minor burns and abrasions.

Although aloe is best known as a topical treatment for injuries to the skin, it also has potent therapeutic effects when taken internally. It has an established role in Chinese medicine, where it is used to clear excessive heat from the liver. It plays a similar detoxifying role in Ayurveda, Tibetan medicine, and other traditional healing cultures across the globe.

BOTANICAL AND PHYTOCHEMICAL INFORMATION

The fleshy leaves of aloe vera are easily recognized by their spiny margins. Individual leaves may be up to a foot and a half long, and each plant may have more than two dozen leaves. The aloe vera plant can be easily propagated by separating a small cluster of leaves that have rooted and replanting them in loose soil.

An aloe vera leaf has three layers, including an outer thick skin, an inner lining, and a central pulp of gel-containing cells. A very bitter, dark yellow juice is obtained from the inner lining, which contains several anthraquinone chemicals that have a strong laxative effect. The gel of the leaf is used topically and internally for its antibiotic and wound healing properties. Aloe vera juice, readily available in health-food stores, is essentially the gel diluted with water.

Many other chemical compounds are found in aloe, including glycosides, steroids, vitamins, and minerals. One chemical constituent of aloe, called acemannan, has been shown to activate immune function, interrupt viral replication, and reduce inflammation.

THE SCIENCE OF ALOE VERA

Aloe vera is best known and most widely studied for its ability to promote wound healing. Serious scientific interest in aloe dates back to the mid 1930s, when it was reported to relieve the smoldering skin inflammation in a woman who had radiation damage to her forehead.[1] Within a day of applying fresh aloe gel, her symptoms improved, and within five months her skin irritation healed fully. Subsequent reports have suggested that the therapeutic effect of aloe may be related to its ability to stimulate the turnover of collagen in the skin, facilitating faster wound repair.[2]

Acting as an inhibitor of prostaglandin chemicals, aloe has potent anti-inflammatory effects when used both orally and topically.[3] In addition to its ability to cool inflammation, aloe has antibiotic activity against both bacteria and fungi. The combination of these properties contributes to its efficacy in enhancing recovery from burn injuries. A recent report found that patients on a burn unit treated with aloe gel healed in less than two-thirds of the time of those whose wounds were treated in the customary manner.[4] Aloe cream has been used successfully in the treatment of psoriasis, with more than 80 percent of patients in a Swedish study reporting substantial benefit.[5] The widespread benefits of aloe in the treatment of tissue injury were demonstrated in a study on frostbite in which aloe showed an ability to limit permanent damage and speed recovery.[6]

Aloe may have value in the prevention and treatment of cancer, although this application is in the preliminary stages of investigation.[7] Potentially valuable uses for aloe vera include its role in the treatment of inflammatory bowel disease and chronic fatigue syndrome. The anti-inflammatory properties of acemannan, a component of aloe vera, may pacify the autoimmune process that damages the digestive tract in ulcerative colitis.[8] Aloe vera may also play a part in a holistic approach to the treatment of chronic fatigue syndrome, a common and debilitating illness for which modern medicine has few effective interventions.[9]

Aloe vera's role in the digestive tract has been studied for many years. Aloin, the chemical component responsible for aloe's laxative effect, was identified in the mid-1800s. In small amounts it helps tone the intestines, but becomes cathartic at higher doses. Although it can be helpful in constipation, it has an irritating effect on the bowel and is not recommended for regular usage. The soothing inner gel contains chemical components that are effective in reducing stomach acid and treating peptic ulcers.[10]

THE PRACTICAL USE OF ALOE VERA

Many traditional properties ascribed to aloe have not yet received scientific attention. In both Chinese and Ayurvedic medicine, aloe is used to help smooth menstrual-cycle concerns, including premenstrual mood swings, bloating, and breast tenderness. It is also reported helpful in reducing the hot flashes of menopause. Aloe has been recommended in the treatment of other hormonal imbalances, including hyperthyroidism and pituitary conditions.

We use aloe vera juice liberally at the Chopra Center. It is a standard component of our detoxification program, in which we encourage people to consume half an ounce of juice twice daily. For people with inflammatory imbalances such as hepatitis, heartburn, skin rashes, emotional irritability, and inflammatory arthritis, we encourage people to take one to two ounces of aloe vera juice three times a day. For teenagers with acne, two ounces of aloe juice mixed into four ounces of carrot juice can help reduce their aggravated skin.

Topically, we routinely recommend aloe gel for stubborn skin irritations. The combination of turmeric powder mixed with aloe and applied directly to insect bites, burns, or acne sores can facilitate rapid healing. Blended with dried lavender flowers, cumin, and comfrey, aloe gel makes a nice facial mask that replenishes dry skin and improves tone.

We rarely use aloe vera powder for its laxative effect. Other herbal cathartics, including senna and cascara sagrada, are equally effective and do not cause as much cramping as aloe.

HOW TO USE ALOE VERA

Aloe vera juice is readily available at health-food stores. We recommend pure aloe vera without other herbal additives. The usual dosage is one-half to two ounces, mixed in apple or cranberry juice, two to three times per day. Fresh aloe gel can be obtained by splitting a leaf with a knife and scraping the gel. We caution against taking homemade gel internally, as it is not always easy to separate the bitter cathartic component from the inner soothing gel.

AYURVEDA AND ALOE VERA

According to Ayurveda, aloe is a complex herb that has bitter, sweet, and pungent flavors with an overall cooling influence on the physiology. Used to cleanse the liver of excessive Pitta while toning digestive power, it is a gentle yet powerful detoxifying substance that is balancing to all three doshas. It is commonly mixed with other substances such as cranberry or pomegranate juice to enhance its purifying properties. Aloe vera juice mixed with raw sugar is used as a general rejuvenative tonic for women transitioning through their menopause.

PRECAUTIONS

Powdered aloe vera obtained from the inner lining of the leaf is strongly laxative and can create bowel laziness. Aloe vera juice derived from the gel is generally safe in usual doses. We do not recommend its internal use during pregnancy.

Circulatory/Respiratory	Detoxifier	Digestive	Immune Enhancer	Men's Health
	X	X		
Metabolic	Nervine	Rejuvenative	Rheumatic	Women's Health
				X

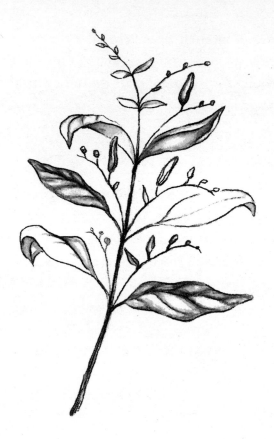

ANDROGRAPHIS
PANICULATA

FAMILIAR: **Indian gentian,
king of bitters**
LATIN: *Andrographis paniculata*
SANSKRIT: kirata, kalmegha,
bhunimb, mahatikta

Thousands of years ago, the Kiratas, a small tribe of people living in the forests of the Himalayan Mountains, utilized a bitter herb to treat fevers. The earliest Ayurvedic sages named this plant *kirata tikta,* meaning the bitter herb of the Kirata people. It was used for the treatment of a wide range of infectious diseases and to clear excessive heat from the liver. During their occupation of India, the British military and administrative forces used this plant, which they called Indian gentian, to treat malaria. Modern scientific studies have confirmed the detoxifying and anti-infectious properties of this ancient remedy.

BOTANICAL AND PHYTOCHEMICAL INFORMATION

Indian gentian is an annual tropical shrub that grows wild throughout the plains of India. It has characteristic four-sided stalks giving rise to three-inch-long pointed leaves. Delicate pink to purplish flowers arise on thin stems and produce small encapsulated fruits containing six to twelve flattened seeds. The entire plant is used medicinally.

A variety of terpenes and flavonoids have been identified in kirata, including several unique compounds called andrographolides. These chemicals appear to be responsible for many of the immunological and circulatory actions of Indian gentian, although some studies have reported that the whole-leaf extract has protective effects on the liver that is not fully accounted for by the andrographolide component.[1]

THE SCIENCE OF INDIAN GENTIAN

Scientific research on Indian gentian has focused on its immune-enhancing and circulatory activity. It has received a lot of attention since the recent publication of a Swedish study that reported a significant benefit of kirata in reducing the symptoms of the common cold.[2] Compared with those taking a placebo, people given Indian gentian showed a faster recovery from the cold, less severe symptoms, and less time missed from work. Earlier studies from Asia and Latin America suggested similar benefits.

Laboratory studies on Indian gentian have demonstrated a variety of pharmacological effects. Mice given extracts of kirata show enhancement of their immune systems, with more aggressive antibody production and cellular responsivity.[3] Although Indian gentian does not appear to have a direct antibacterial effect, it may confer protection from a wide range of infections including malaria, parasites, and retroviruses.[4-7] People with tonsillitis experience more rapid relief of their fever and sore throat, and patients who undergo treatment for kidney stones have fewer urinary tract infections.[8, 9] Early clinical trials in HIV-infected men have suggested that an Indian gentian extract may lead to modest improvements in immune function.[10] Although these findings are limited,

they do provide the impetus for further scientific study into the immune-enhancing potential of Indian gentian.

Another potentially important role for Indian gentian is in the treatment of heart disease. Studies in animals have shown it to have a wide range of physiological effects that may benefit people with coronary heart problems. Indian gentian has blood-pressure-lowering and heart-rate-slowing effects, both of which can reduce the strain on oxygen-deficient heart muscle.[11] In studies of animals with heart attacks, Indian gentian reduces the damage to heart tissue and the frequency of life-threatening irregularities in the heart rhythm.[12] Several reports in both animals and people have confirmed kirata's ability to reduce the stickiness of platelets, which has the effect of reducing undesirable blood vessel clotting.[13, 14] A study in China tested the combined benefit of these different properties in dogs fed a high-cholesterol diet.[15] After their severely obstructed blood vessels were opened by angioplasty, those who were given Indian gentian had much milder reblockage despite continuing a high-fat diet. Such findings warrant further studies to see if these benefits are applicable to people with heart disease.

Kirata has traditionally been used to protect the liver, and several studies have provided scientific support for this role. Animals given Indian gentian along with chemicals known to be toxic to the liver have much less liver damage.[16, 17] In one study, Indian gentian was more effective than silymarin (milk thistle) in protecting the liver.[18] In addition to an antioxidant effect, kirata stimulates the flow of bile, which could be helpful in the prevention of bile stones.[19] In view of its long history in Ayurveda and encouraging laboratory studies, Indian gentian is deserving of further research to see what role it may play in the prevention and treatment of liver disease.

THE PRACTICAL USE OF INDIAN GENTIAN

Indian gentian is just beginning to be noticed in the West, despite its use for over a decade in Scandinavian countries. In addition to its importance in the Ayurvedic herbal pharmacy, it is valued by Chinese medicine, where it is known as chuan xin lian. It is not yet readily available as a single herb, but is a component of many immune-enhancing formulas.

For the treatment of viral upper respiratory symptoms, it usually is taken at the earliest sign of symptoms and continued for one week. As an aid in a detoxification program, it should be taken at most for two weeks, unless a knowledgeable health-care provider prescribes it and is monitoring you. Preliminary studies in HIV-infected patients reported positive laboratory findings within six weeks of beginning the herb.[20] If you are going to use it for this condition, be sure to work closely with your health-care adviser so that you can carefully monitor your viral counts and immune function.

HOW TO USE INDIAN GENTIAN

When treating the symptoms of a cold or flu, the dose used in published studies is 340 milligrams three times daily for five days. The available products in the West usually are standardized to 10 percent andrographolides. About the same dosage was used initially in the HIV studies (5 milligrams per kilogram of body weight three times daily) and was then increased (10 to 20 mg/kg) during the course of six weeks. Indian gentian is also available in herbal extracts recommended for sore throats and colds.

AYURVEDA AND INDIAN GENTIAN

Indian gentian is very bitter in taste and has a drying, cooling influence on the physiology. It is pacifying to Pitta and Kapha, but can be aggravating to Vata. It is traditionally used in conditions of Pitta aggravation in which a person has excessive heat congestion attributed to accumulated liver toxicity.

PRECAUTIONS

Indian gentian has a detoxifying effect and can be depleting if used for a prolonged time. Animal studies have suggested that kirata has anti-fertility properties in both males and females.[20] Although this effect has not been reported in people, those trying to get pregnant are best to avoid it. It is also contraindicated in pregnancy.

Circulatory/Respiratory	Detoxifier	Digestive	Immune Enhancer	Men's Health
X	X	X	X	
Metabolic	Nervine	Rejuvenative	Rheumatic	Women's Health

ASPARAGUS RACEMOSUS

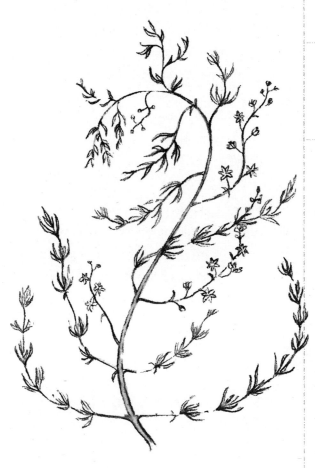

FAMILIAR: **wild asparagus**
LATIN: *Asparagus racemosus*
SANSKRIT: shatavari

Shatavari is one of the prime rejuvenating herbal medicines in Ayurveda. It is considered particularly helpful in conditions affecting the female reproductive system. One of its names means "having one hundred roots," which bespeaks its reputation as a fertility-enhancing plant.

A member of the same family as the common asparagus, shatavari has nutritive properties. Commonly used in India to improve the production of breast milk in nursing mothers, it is even fed to cows to enhance their milk output. It is also effective in relieving inflammatory conditions and in soothing irritated tissues.

BOTANICAL AND PHYTOCHEMICAL INFORMATION

Shatavari's native home is in the lowland jungles of India. The asparagus plant is a natural climber that is commonly cultivated in Indian gardens. It produces small, white, fragrant flowers and red berries, but it is the roots and succulent tubers that are used as both food and medicine.

Active saponins, which are chemically extracted from shatavari using alcohol or ether, have the effect of suppressing uterine contractions. Water extracts of shatavari have been shown to reduce the growth of various microorganisms.

THE SCIENCE OF SHATAVARI

There has been relatively little scientific research into shatavari, despite its long-standing reputation as a valuable tonic. Studies in the 1960s explored its role as a milk promoter in animals.[1, 2] Although preliminary studies suggested that it could increase breast milk production in buffalo and rats, a recent controlled investigation in lactating women did not find any difference between those consuming shatavari and those taking a placebo.[3]

Its traditional role as a digestive aid has received some scientific support. In men with a history of heartburn and indigestion after meals, shatavari was found to be as effective as metoclopramide, a pharmaceutical agent commonly used to treat nausea.[4] Although it has not been formally studied, shatavari also has an established history as an anti-diarrhea agent.

The immune-modulating properties of shatavari have received the most scientific attention. Shatavari has a measurable effect on the functioning of macrophages. These important immune cells are responsible for digesting potentially harmful organisms as well as cancer cells. Studies on shatavari have shown that it can enhance the ability of macrophages to do their job against the fungus candida.[5] Shatavari helps the immune system recover more quickly after it has been exposed to toxic chemicals, both by enhancing the production of natural immune-regulating messenger molecules and by protecting blood-producing cells in the bone marrow.[6, 7] Shatavari's various effects on the immune system have been shown to reduce the development of scar tissue after surgery in animals.[8] All of these properties may have important clinical applications in people, but more research is needed to determine whether the laboratory findings are relevant to humans.

THE PRACTICAL USE OF SHATAVARI

Shatavari is described in Ayurveda as having a nourishing, smoothing, cooling, lubricating influence on the physiology. As such, it is used in conditions when the body and mind are overheated, depleted, or out of balance. It is commonly recommended for women who are having menstrual problems, particularly when irritability and mood swings are prominent. Its cooling influence may also benefit the hot flashes of women going through menopause. Shatavari is beneficial in cooling off an irritated digestive system as expressed by heartburn, diarrhea, or irritable bowel syndrome. It can also be helpful to soothe irritation in the urinary tract.

Its nutritive properties are invaluable in people recovering from illness, particularly when there has been substantial weight loss. Shatavari has a reputation as an enhancer of fertility. It is said to increase the health of both male and female reproductive tissue.

How to Use Shatavari

Shatavari is now available in the United States in both powdered and capsule forms. When used to treat digestive distress, one teaspoon in one-half cup of warm milk is taken after each meal. It mixes well with equal parts of amalaki and licorice for symptoms of heartburn or indigestion. For symptoms of PMS or menopausal hot flashes, 500-milligram capsules can be used in doses up to 2 grams per day.

A teaspoon of powdered shatavari mixed with brown sugar and organic milk can be added to the diet several times per day in anyone recovering from a debilitating illness or surgery. Taken in cool water, shatavari can be used to treat the irritation associated with nonspecific urethritis or interstitial cystitis, two conditions that modern medicine treats with difficulty.

Ayurveda and Shatavari

Shatavari is sweet and bitter in taste. It is balancing to Pitta and Vata, and in excess can mildly increase Kapha. It is one of the primary rasayanas of value for both men and women.

Precautions

Although it is traditionally recommended for lactating mothers, we have not come across any studies that have evaluated its safety. It is closely related to the common asparagus, and we would not anticipate serious health concerns arising from its use by breastfeeding mothers. Its rich qualities can occasionally aggravate sinus congestion in people with Kapha tendencies.

Circulatory/Respiratory	Detoxifier	Digestive	Immune Enhancer	Men's Health
		X	X	
Metabolic	Nervine	Rejuvenative	Rheumatic	Women's Health
		X		X

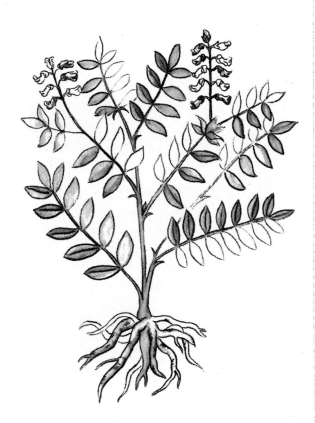

ASTRAGALUS MEMBRANECEUS

FAMILIAR: **astragalus, milk vetch, yellow vetch**
LATIN: *Astragalus membraneceus*
CHINESE: huang qi

Astragalus membraneceus, one of the most important tonics in traditional Chinese medicine, is just beginning to gain popularity in the West. Often considered the counterpart of ginseng, astragalus has long been used in Asia to enhance vital energy and strengthen the defensive forces of the body. Recent scientific studies have documented profound immune-enhancing properties of astragalus that may be of therapeutic value in the treatment of illnesses ranging from cancer to autoimmune diseases.

BOTANICAL AND PHYTOCHEMICAL INFORMATION

The *Astragalus* genus of plants includes almost 2,500 hundred species, making it the largest on earth. Astragalus is a member of the legume or pea family, but it is the roots that are the source of the prized herbal medicine. A perennial plant that grows to a height of about one and one-half feet, astragalus is native to eastern China and Mongolia. The dense bushy leaves composed of a dozen paired leaflets give rise to purple pea-like flowers. The roots of plants several years old are harvested, dried, and made into powders and tinctures.

A number of chemical constituents have been identified in astragalus roots, including polysaccharides, triterpenoids, isoflavones, choline, and saponins. Several unique compounds called astragalosides have been isolated. The chemicals responsible for the various pharmacological actions of astragalus have not been fully characterized; however, the polysaccharides and saponins are the most likely candidates for its immune-modulating properties.

THE SCIENCE OF ASTRAGALUS

Dozens of studies in both animals and people have demonstrated dramatic effects of astragalus on the immune system. Different experiments have tested the protective effect of astragalus on the immune system by giving animals an immune-suppressing drug or radiation. In many studies the administration of astragalus partially or completely reversed the effects of the toxic intervention on the bone marrow and lymph system.[1, 2] Other studies have shown that astragalus can stimulate immune cells to respond to a variety of challenges more aggressively, resulting in a slowing of cancer cell growth and viral replication.[3, 4]

One of the nasty secrets of cancer cells is their ability to secrete chemicals that have the effect of sedating immune cells. This immune depression reduces the ability of the body to identify and eliminate malignant cells. Laboratory studies have shown that taking suppressed immune cells and incubating them with astragalus helps substantially to restore their potency.[5, 6]

Modern cancer researchers are increasingly looking to nature for ways to fight this dreaded disease. A developing class of medicines known as biological response modifiers makes use of the natural disease fighting chemicals of the body. One of these substances, interleukin-2 (IL-2) has been shown to be a powerful weapon in certain types of cancer. Unfortunately, it also has powerful side effects, limiting the amount that can be safely tolerated by cancer patients. A laboratory study from Texas found that astragalus potentiated the tumor-cell-killing effect of IL-2, allowing for lower doses to be used without a loss of efficacy.[7] If this can be shown to be applicable to people, astragalus could play a valuable role in future cancer treatment protocols.

The clinical application of these laboratory findings has been tested in a group of patients with lung cancer who received astragalus along with standard radiation and chemotherapy. Those receiving the immune-enhancing herb had significantly improved rates of survival, even in patients with more-advanced stages of illness.[8] The potential of astragalus to improve the outcome of people with cancer is worthy of further exploration.

Astragalus may provide value in the treatment of other health concerns. Patients with the autoimmune disease systemic lupus erythematosus (SLE) are susceptible to infections, despite their aggravated immune state. A study from China found that their immune cells were usually unable to respond normally to challenges, but the addition of astragalus could improve their function.[9] Astragalus has also been reported to enhance immunity in people suffering with viral infections of the heart, a rare but potentially disabling condition.[10]

The role of astragalus on other heart conditions has received attention, with several reports suggesting it can improve function and reduce the symptoms of people with coronary heart disease. Heart patients given astragalus have shown fewer episodes of anginal chest pain, improvement in their EKGs, and healthier cardiac function.[11, 12] A laboratory study reported that astragalus improved the utilization of oxygen by heart cells.[13] The investigation of astragalus in the treatment of heart disease, the most common serious health problem of our society, is a worthy scientific pursuit. Preliminary reports of the benefit of astragalus on memory, infertility, and protection from liver damage highlight the diverse potential benefits of this ancient healing herb.[14–16]

THE PRACTICAL USE OF ASTRAGALUS

As a rejuvenative, astragalus can be valuable for people who do not have the energy they desire. It is particularly useful for those who feel their circulation is weak because they frequently have cold hands and feet.

As an immune-enhancing agent it seems to have a sustained benefit, unlike echinacea, which tends to lose its efficacy after a couple of weeks. If you are facing a serious health challenge such as cancer, discuss the use of astragalus as an immune tonic with your doctor. It can also be used at the onset of a cold or flu to boost your body's defenses.

Its role in heart disease is less clearly defined, although reports have suggested it can be valuable in both acute and chronic cardiac conditions. If you are under treatment for a heart ailment, be sure to discuss the use of astragalus or any other medicinal substance with your health-care provider before adding it to your regimen.

HOW TO USE ASTRAGALUS

Astragalus is now readily available through health-food stores. It is usually found in capsules of 400 to 500 milligrams of the dried root. Extracts and tinctures are also available, in which astragalus is usually combined with tonic Chinese herbs. Tea bags containing astragalus are coming to the health-food market.

For general immune enhancement, take 2 to 4 grams daily in divided doses. If you can find dried astragalus root at an Asian food or herb store, simmer a heaping tablespoon for ten minutes, strain, and drink a cup two or three times per day.

AYURVEDA AND ASTRAGALUS

Not described by the original sages, astragalus can be understood in Ayurvedic terms. The root is predominantly sweet in taste with a warming potency. Astragalus is a valuable rejuvenative for all doshas and is particularly balancing for Vata. In excess, it can mildly increase Kapha and Pitta.

PRECAUTIONS

Astragalus has a long safety record. We have not encountered any accounts from the traditional or scientific literature of adverse reactions attributed to it. Theoretically, its immune-enhancing effect could be aggravating to autoimmune conditions, although none have been reported.

Circulatory/Respiratory	Detoxifier	Digestive	Immune Enhancer	Men's Health
X			X	
Metabolic	Nervine	Rejuvenative	Rheumatic	Women's Health
		X		

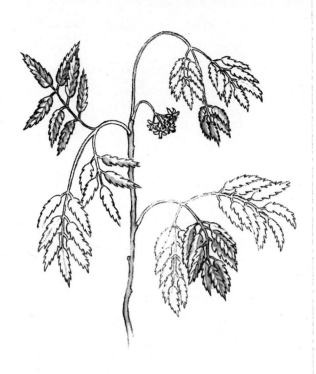

AZADIRACHTA INDICA

FAMILIAR: **neem, margosa, Persian lilac**
LATIN: *Azadirachta indica*
SANSKRIT: nimba, arishta

The neem tree, native to India, is revered as its own botanical pharmacy, providing leaves, seed oil, and bark with a wide range of healing benefits. This beautiful evergreen tree is highly resistant to insects and infections, which alerted ancient healers to its disease-resistant properties. Traditionally, neem was taken internally as a blood purifier and detoxifying agent in patients with chronic fevers and infections. Ayurvedic medicine considers neem to be especially effective as a medicated oil for the treatment of skin infections, inflammatory skin conditions, joint pain, and muscle aches. In rural areas of India, twigs of the neem tree are used as toothbrushes to strengthen the gums and prevent gingivitis.

BOTANICAL AND PHYTOCHEMICAL INFORMATION

Chemical analysis of neem flowers, leaves, seeds, and bark have identified a variety of bitter substances, some of which are unique to this tree. Nimbin and azadirachtin have been identified as bitter components of neem tree bark and seeds that may confer disease resistance. Antifungal, antibacterial, and antimalarial activity have been documented for extracts derived from neem leaves and seeds. Neem is also widely used as a component of nontoxic insecticides and has been the recent subject of international controversy as Western pesticide companies seek patents for effective chemical compounds identified in neem.

THE SCIENCE OF NEEM

Neem has traditionally been used to treat infections, diabetes, obesity, anxiety, and pain. It is also reputed to protect the liver against toxic injuries caused by drugs or viruses. Modern studies have suggested that many of the properties traditionally attributed to neem can be scientifically validated. Extracts of neem have been shown to inhibit bacterial, fungal, and parasitic infections.[1, 2] In addition to a direct effect on potentially harmful organisms, neem also enhances several aspects of immune function.[3] A recent report from the UCLA School of Dentistry found that neem could reduce the ability of streptococcal bacteria to colonize the surface of teeth, providing an explanation for neem's long-standing reputation as a cavity fighter.[4] A neem and turmeric paste applied to the scalp is very effective for the treatment of scabies, a common and contagious skin infection caused by a tiny mite.[5] In tropical countries, neem's antibiotic properties are applied for the treatment of malaria and to curtail mosquito growth.

Neem has been shown to have measurable anti-inflammatory actions, anti-anxiety effects, and significant pain relieving properties.[6, 7, 8] A potentially important clinical benefit of neem is its ability to reduce the incidence of stomach ulcers in response to stress by blunting the release of inflammatory chemicals.[9] Although its efficacy in human beings is yet to be fully documented, neem has been shown to lower blood sugar levels in animals, giving support to one of its traditional roles as an anti-diabetes herb.[10]

Neem has been shown to have contraceptive and abortifacient effects in animal studies, which may eventually have practical applications in people.[11, 12] Because of these properties, neem products should not be taken by women who are or may be pregnant.

THE PRACTICAL USE OF NEEM

We prescribe neem when we believe a person needs gentle detoxification. People who have been overeating, abusing drugs or alcohol, or who have recently taken steroids, antibiotics, or cancer chemotherapy drugs benefit from the cleansing effect of neem. People attempting to lose weight and those facing Type II diabetes mellitus may also be helped by the toxin-reducing properties of neem.

Externally, neem is useful for inflammatory skin lesions such as allergic dermatitis or eczema. It can also be directly applied to acne skin lesions. If someone appears to have toxic accumulations but is quite debilitated, we use neem cautiously, as it has a depleting effect on tissues.

HOW TO USE NEEM

Neem leaves are available in Indian and Middle Eastern food stores, where they are sold as a culinary spice. Neem leaves added to soups, casseroles, or vegetable dishes add a pleasant bitter flavor and serve to reduce toxic accumulations. Neem powder and neem oil are available at most health-food stores. If you are using neem as a detoxifying agent, take one-half teaspoon in juice or water three times daily for one week. If you are using neem topically for a skin infection, make a paste with neem powder and apply it twice daily. For dry, irritated skin, apply medicated neem oil twice daily until the area clears.

Neem trees are now readily available from farms where they can be grown in climates where it does not freeze, such as Florida or Southern California. Whether you are able to pick the leaves off your tree or obtain them from an Indian market, try steeping them in hot water, then spraying the infusion on fruit or vegetable plants to limit insect and fungal infestations. Neem leaves have been used for centuries to protect clothing and papers from mold and mildew. According to Ayurveda, neem should be included in everyone's home pharmacy.

AYURVEDA AND NEEM

From an Ayurvedic perspective, neem is bitter, drying, and cold, making it a useful medicinal herb in conditions that are hot and damp. It can be helpful in Kapha and Pitta conditions, but may exacerbate Vata problems. Its drying and purifying qualities contribute to neem's role in inflammatory and toxic states. Neem's detoxifying properties also explain its value in problems of retention and excess, such as diabetes and obesity.

PRECAUTIONS

Due to its contraceptive and possible abortion-promoting properties, neem should be avoided in woman of childbearing years who are pregnant or may want to become pregnant. It should also be used cautiously in people who are severely depleted from chronic illness or poor nutrition.

Circulatory/Respiratory	Detoxifier	Digestive	Immune Enhancer	Men's Health
	X		X	
Metabolic	Nervine	Rejuvenative	Rheumatic	Women's Health
X			X	

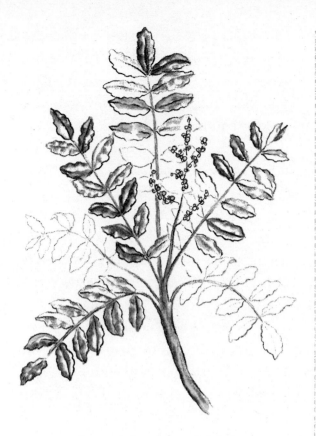

BOSWELLIA
SERRATA

FAMILIAR: **boswellia, Indian olibanum, salai guggal**
LATIN: *Boswellia serrata*
SANSKRIT: shallaki, kunduru

Boswellia is also known as Indian frankincense, one of several plants in a family of resinous trees famous for their aromatic oils. Prized from North Africa to India, frankincense, along with myrrh and gold, was among the original offerings to the Christ Child. Referenced in the earliest Ayurvedic texts, boswellia was traditionally used to treat respiratory ailments, disorders of the digestive system, and joint diseases. Pharmacological studies performed in the late 1960s and early 1970s identified unique pain-relieving, sedating, and anti-inflammatory properties in extracts of boswellia. Clinical studies are now confirming many of the traditional uses for boswellia, including the treatment of asthma, arthritis, and inflammatory bowel diseases.

BOTANICAL AND PHYTOCHEMICAL INFORMATION

Many closely related trees yield the fragrant resin known as frankincense. Boswellia trees are native to North Africa and the Middle East, but it is only in the dry, mountainous forests of western and central India that *Boswellia serrata* can be found. The tree, which can grow slowly to eighteen feet in height, has a thick, papery bark that yields a gummy exudate when peeled away or cut.

The gum contains a variety of natural sugars, volatile essential oils, and terpenoids. Several unique triterpene acids, identified in the terpenoid component, have been named *boswellic acids* and appear to account for boswellia's medicinal properties. Animal studies on the alcoholic extract of the gum have demonstrated potent anti-inflammatory actions by inhibiting the production of prostaglandins.[1]

THE SCIENCE OF BOSWELLIA

Prostaglandin chemicals play an important role in many different physiological functions. They are essential in the regulation of the digestive, respiratory, and urinary tracts. They also play a pivotal role in the clotting system and are the fundamental chemical messengers in an inflammatory response. Boswellia has been shown to inhibit an important enzyme in the formation of inflammatory prostaglandins, known as 5-lipoxygenase.[2, 3] The blocking of this enzyme reduces the production of chemicals called leukotrienes, which provoke and perpetuate inflammation.[4, 5]

Excessive production of leukotrienes has been implicated in a variety of immune disorders including asthma, rheumatoid arthritis, and ulcerative colitis. Boswellia has been shown to provide potential therapeutic benefits in each of these health conditions. In a recent paper from Germany, 70 percent of patients with bronchial asthma who received boswellia showed improvement in their breathing, compared with only 27 percent of those given a placebo.[6] The benefits were apparent clinically as well as through breathing and blood studies.

Boswellia has classically been used in the treatment of joint pain and inflammation. Animal studies have shown boswellia to reduce the deterioration of joint sugars and proteins required for healthy function.[7] People taking boswellia along with ashwagandha, turmeric, and zinc for degenerative osteoarthritis reported less joint pain, better movement, and improved strength without any serious side effects.[8] Although case reports have suggested that boswellia is also beneficial in rheumatoid arthritis, a recent German report did not find any difference between those taking the herb and those on a placebo, although over half of the patients did not complete the study.[9]

Leukotrienes have been implicated in the smoldering inflammation associated with ulcerative colitis, an inflammatory bowel disorder that affects about one in one thousand people. A study from India that compared the use of boswellia with the standard drug treatment for ulcerative colitis found that 82 percent of patients taking the herb went into remission, compared with 75 percent on the medication.[10] A wide range of measurements improved, including the frequency of bowel movements and the microscopic findings on biopsies.

Although these studies in people are limited, it is encouraging that this apparently safe and inexpensive herb can provide such a wide range of potential benefits. It may be very rewarding for medical research to explore the potential value of boswellia in the many inflammatory conditions that afflict people.

THE PRACTICAL USE OF BOSWELLIA

From an Ayurvedic perspective, boswellia is useful in the treatment of an expansive variety of health concerns. It is said to have stimulating properties, can help mobilize phlegm in respiratory conditions, and treats digestive disturbances, from heartburn to diarrhea. It is part of several Ayurvedic obesity formulas, in which it is said to enhance metabolic activity. As a paste, boswellia can be applied directly to skin irritations ranging from diabetic ulcers to acne. As a cream or poultice applied to joints, it can reduce the pain of arthritis and injury.

Boswellia can normalize menstrual irregularities and treat liver ailments. It has been used traditionally to treat both syphilis and gonorrhea. As a mouthwash, it can treat bad breath due to gum disease. If there is a common theme to the traditional role of boswellia, it is its purported efficacy in conditions of excessive inflammation.

HOW TO USE BOSWELLIA

Boswellia is now widely available in the West from a variety of herbal companies. Most doses are standardized to contain between 37.5 and 65 percent boswellic acids, yielding 150 to 200 milligrams per tablet or capsule. Check the information on the bottle to determine whether the dosing is in terms of the herb compound or the boswellic acid extract. For example, a 300-milligram tablet standardized to yield 65 percent boswellic acids will provide 195 milligrams of boswellic acids. Studies have used daily doses between 450 milligrams (150 milligrams three times a day) and 1,200 milligrams (400 milligrams three times a day).

Boswellia is also available as a component of a topical cream, combined with capsaicin and salycilates. This can be applied to sore muscles and aching joints several times daily.

AYURVEDA AND BOSWELLIA

According to Ayurveda, boswellia carries the astringent, bitter, and sweet tastes. It has a cooling effect on the physiology. It is most pacifying to Pitta and can also reduce Kapha. It is mildly aggravating to Vata in high doses.

PRECAUTIONS

Unlike most anti-inflammatory medications, boswellia is not reported to cause stomach ulcers or gastritis. People rarely report mild nausea, diarrhea, or a skin rash.

Circulatory/Respiratory	Detoxifier	Digestive	Immune Enhancer	Men's Health
X		X		
Metabolic	Nervine	Rejuvenative	Rheumatic	Women's Health
X			X	

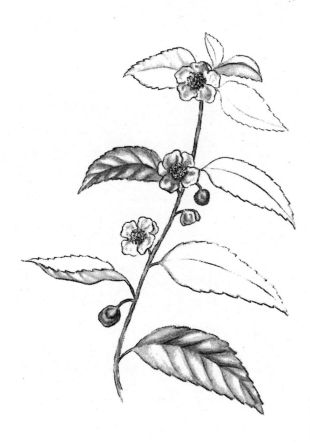

CAMELLIA SINENSIS

FAMILIAR: **tea**
LATIN: *Camellia sinensis, Thea sinensis*
SANSKRIT/HINDI: chai

Other than water, tea is consumed by more people than any other beverage on earth. Tea has been a part of the human diet for close to five thousand years, since its discovery by the legendary Chinese emperor Shen Nong. The story goes that he stopped with his entourage for refreshment, and while his cook was boiling water, the leaves of a nearby bush blew into the water, resulting in the first herbal infusion of what we now call tea.

This invigorating herb from China spread to Japan and India, then across Europe and Russia. Arriving in the New World in the late seventeenth century, tea became the symbol of the struggle between independence-minded colonists and their British oppressors, sparking the revolution that birthed the United States. Tea has always had the tendency to arouse passions.

Although prized for its astringent taste and refreshing energy boost, tea has also been long valued for its medicinal properties. It has been used to settle the digestive system, treat infections, soothe pain, and overcome fatigue. Recent scientific studies have documented tea's health-promoting effects in conditions ranging from dental cavities to cancer.

BOTANICAL AND PHYTOCHEMICAL INFORMATION

The bush from which we obtain tea leaves can grow wild to thirty feet in height, but the cultivated evergreen plants are usually trimmed to stand below six feet. The finer teas use only the two young top leaves and bud. Green tea leaves are picked and allowed to wither in the hot air, then pan-fried to stop the fermentation process. Oolong tea is derived from leaves that are shaken and bruised and allowed to partially oxidize until the edges of the leaves turn red. Black teas are allowed to ferment in cool, humid rooms until the entire leaf darkens. These different processes alter both the flavor and chemical content of the teas.

Tea leaves contain many compounds including flavonoids, polysaccharides, and various vitamins, but it is the polyphenols that seem to be the most potent therapeutic phytochemicals. Originally known as tea tannins, polyphenols make up about one-quarter of fresh dried green tea leaves. The polyphenols in tea are known as catechins, and include gallocatechin, epigallocatechin, epicatechin, epicatechin gallate, and epigallocatechin gallate (EGCG). These catechins are potent antioxidants and appear to play a role in protecting the body from cancer and cardiovascular diseases. The EGCG polyphenol component comprises almost sixty percent of the total catechins present in tea and seems to have the greatest health promoting impact. The darker the tea, the lower the content of antioxidizing polyphenols available in the leaves.

THE SCIENCE OF TEA

One cup of tea has the antioxidant activity of ten glasses of apple juice or three glasses of orange juice.[1] A group from the National Institute of Nutrition in Italy found that the antioxidant capacity of green tea is six times that of black tea.[2] Interestingly, when human subjects took their tea with milk, the antioxidant effect of both the green and black varieties was reduced.

Laboratory studies on tea or tea components have shown potential benefits in the suppression of cancer growth. In mice given carcinogenic chemicals, tea improved their immune cells' ability to identify and eliminate potentially malignant cells.[3] In laboratory cultures of tumor cells, green tea extracts showed potent inhibition of cancer cell growth.[4] Both green and black tea have been found to inhibit DNA reproduction and promote the demise of tumor cells.[5]

Studies looking at the relationship between tea drinkers and cancer in people have generally suggested a protective effect from tea. Japanese women who regularly drank tea before developing breast cancer had significantly reduced recurrences and improved outcomes.[6] The incidence of prostate cancer in Chinese men is the lowest in the world and correlated with their tea intake, suggests that green tea may confer some protection against this common malignancy in men.[7] The risk of colon cancer may be slightly reduced in green tea drinkers, while the risk of lung cancer may be slightly elevated in black tea drinkers who also smoke.[8] Overall, the polyphenols present in green tea seem to have a cancer-protecting effect, although it is not clear how long and how much one has to drink to gain the benefit.

Tea has also been associated with a reduction in coronary heart disease. Animal studies have shown that tea has a mild cholesterol-lowering effect, although this has been harder to demonstrate in people.[9-11] Studies from around the world have suggested that tea drinkers have lower blood pressure and fewer coronary heart attacks, and live longer.[12-14] Not every report has confirmed this advantage, raising the possibility that people who take their tea with milk do not derive the same benefit as those who take their tea alone.[15]

Other therapeutic effects of tea have been reported, including the prevention of dental cavities, accelerated weight loss in dieters, and reduced digestive symptoms in people with inflammatory bowel disease.[16-18] Tea has known antibacterial properties, which are greater in green tea and lesser in black. This may in part explain its traditional use in the treatment of infectious dysentery. In addition to providing refreshment, this ancient herbal brew has many potential therapeutic benefits.

THE PRACTICAL USE OF TEA

Although green tea tablets are now available, the best way to partake of this helpful herb is to savor a cup of tea. Green tea and oolong are usually consumed alone or with a little sweetener, but not with milk or lemon. The blacker the tea, the greater the tendency to add milk, but this may reduce its medicinal value. For a delicious treat, try a cup of masala chai, prepared by mixing cardamom seeds, cloves, fresh ginger, and a black peppercorn with tea and milk. Sweeten to taste for an afternoon pick-me-up.

HOW TO USE TEA

High-quality green, oolong, and black teas are readily available from specialty grocers, coffee shops, and Asian food stores. Although five to six cups of tea a day are often consumed in China and Japan, one or two cups of green tea will provide a hefty dose of polyphenols without charging you up with caffeine.

Use one cup of boiling water per one teaspoon of loose tea, and steep for five minutes before sipping slowly. You can make iced green tea by placing two teaspoons per cup of cold water and brewing the mixture in a closed jar placed in the refrigerator for a couple of hours. Powdered green tea tablets and capsules are available in doses equivalent to up to ten cups of tea, but we prefer the more natural infusion.

AYURVEDA AND TEA

Tea carries the bitter and astringent tastes, and has a cooling influence on the physiology. It is balancing to Pitta and Kapha, but can be aggravating to Vata.

PRECAUTIONS

Adverse reactions to tea are exceedingly rare. Owing to its caffeine content, it can produce nervousness and insomnia in sensitive individuals. The caffeine content differs by the type of tea; green tea (8–36 milligrams) contains less than oolong (12–55 milligrams), which has less than black tea (25–110 milligrams). By comparison, a cup of coffee has 100 to 160 milligrams, while a can of Diet Coke has 46 milligrams of caffeine. Heavy tea drinkers can experience caffeine withdrawal headaches if they suddenly discontinue their intake.

Two medical complications of tea drinking have recently been reported. In one, a sixty-one-year-old woman developed a low potassium blood level leading to irregularities in her heart rate after drinking two to three *liters* of oolong tea per day.[19] In another case, a man taking blood thinners began drinking up to a gallon of green tea on a daily basis. The blood thinning effects of the medication were neutralized, presumably due to the high dose of vitamin K he was receiving from the tea.[20] These are both extreme examples but highlight that even though something is derived from natural sources it can cause problems if used inappropriately. Used in a balanced way, this ancient beverage can be a health-promoting ally.

Circulatory/Respiratory	Detoxifier	Digestive	Immune Enhancer	Men's Health
X			X	
Metabolic	Nervine	Rejuvenative	Rheumatic	Women's Health
X				

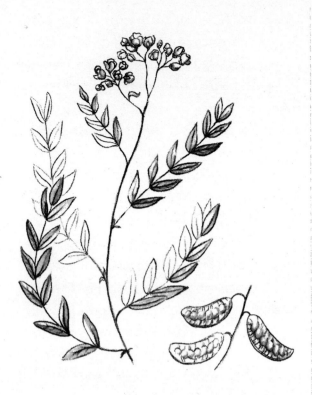

CASSIA
ANGUSTIFOLIA

FAMILIAR: **senna**
LATIN: *Cassia angustifolia, Cassia
acutifolia, Cassia senna*
SANSKRIT: rajavriksha, markandika

With several hundred known species of *Cassia,* traditional medicinal cultures around the world have recognized the potent laxative effects of senna. Native to northern Africa, senna is now grown on most continents and is one of the most popular bowel agents in the world. Used appropriately, senna is an effective bowel stimulant that can get sluggish bowels moving without serious side effects. However, if you feel the need to use a laxative on a regular basis, look to your diet for ways to improve your digestive function before resorting to an herbal stimulant.

Well known to both Ayurveda and traditional Chinese medicine, senna's traditional therapeutic properties have extended beyond its actions on the digestive tract. In Ayurveda, senna has been used in the treatment of chronic inflammatory skin disorders, premenstrual symptoms, and high blood pressure. In traditional Chinese medicine, senna is useful in balancing excessive heat in the liver and as a treatment for cardiovascular disorders.

BOTANICAL
AND PHYTOCHEMICAL
INFORMATION

The medicinal herb is derived from the dried leaves or pods of this three-foot high bushy plant. Stems have between five and ten pairs of leaves and small yellow flowers. The slightly curved pods are harvested in the fall. The powdered pods produce a gentler laxative response than the leaves.

The laxative effect of senna is due to its content of anthraquinone chemicals, which stimulate the digestive tract to contract and alter the transport of fluids and salts across the intestinal lining. The primary anthraquinones identified in senna are named sennoside A and B. These are closely related to similar compounds found in castor oil, the latex of aloe vera, rhubarb, and *Cascara sagrada*. Anthraquinones present in herbal products are converted into active ingredients by normal bacteria in the colon. Once activated, these chemicals have complex effects on intestinal cells, resulting in the accumulation of salts and water in the gut and the stimulation of colonic movement.[1]

THE SCIENCE OF SENNA

Senna is a moderately potent herbal laxative that has predictable effects on the digestive tract. Ingested leaves or pods have minimal effects until they reach the large intestines, where normal bacteria metabolize the chemical constituents into active metabolic products. These activated sennosides, called rhine anthrone and sennidins A and B, interact with colon cells, resulting in the release of prostaglandins. These prostaglandins, along with calcium, cause water and salt to be secreted into the colon and stimulate the contraction of intestinal muscle cells.[2] The combined effects result in more-liquid bowel movements. Constipation can be due to inadequate dietary bulk and insufficient fluids. At appropriate doses, senna restores normal consistency to bowel movements by increasing the moisture in the colon, but

when an excessive amount of senna is taken, diarrhea can result.

Several studies have found senna to be a cost-effective treatment for chronic constipation. In studies in elderly patients from both Ireland and Finland, senna significantly improved bowel function with minimal side effects and at lower cost than lactulose, another commonly used bowel agent.[3, 4] Senna has also been found useful for patients with constipation resulting from narcotic medication use. Abdominal discomfort is common in cancer patients because the opiate pain medicines they require often cause a slowdown in digestive function. Senna has been shown to improve bowel function in cancer patients on narcotic medication, but cramping may be a limiting side effect.[5, 6]

People immobilized by illness or injury often experience sluggish bowel function. Studies looking at the value of senna after major surgery and childbirth have found it to be effective, with only minor adverse effects.[7, 8] Senna has also been shown useful in preparing patients for surgery, with greater efficacy and fewer side effects than other standard bowel agents.[9]

When used intermittently, senna is effective and generally well tolerated. An important question is whether or not it is safe to use senna on a consistent basis. Animal studies have shown that taking senna in doses that induce diarrhea will eventually lead to fluid and salt imbalances, and its effectiveness in inducing bowel movements diminishes.[10] Animals do not seem to habituate to senna at the lower doses that stimulate normal-consistency bowel movements. In fact, some reports have suggested that appropriate doses of senna may help to "re-educate" the bowels to function more regularly.[11, 12] Although there may not be any serious complications to using senna on a regular basis, from a holistic perspective we believe that it is preferable to make the necessary diet and lifestyle changes rather than rely on an herbal medicine to sustain a normal physiological function.

Although the bulk of the attention on senna has focused on its obvious digestive effects, studies have suggested that senna has other potentially beneficial health properties. A study in rats found that a close cousin to senna significantly reduced both cholesterol and triglyceride levels without causing any serious negative effects.[13] Other studies have shown that the anthraquinones in senna are potent antioxidants.[14] Finally, both antiviral and antibacterial properties of senna have been demonstrated.[15, 16]

THE PRACTICAL USE OF SENNA

Senna is a component of many digestive herbal products. The most commonly available form of senna is a standardized extract, Sennokot. After ingesting senna, a bowel movement usually occurs within six to twelve hours. A dose taken at bedtime will therefore usually act by the next morning. Some people are more sensitive to senna than others, so if you are a first-time user, allow enough time for it to take effect, or you may find yourself rushing to the bathroom in the middle of an office meeting.

Senna is not recommended for more than one week's use continuously. If you feel the need to use senna, first take an honest inventory of your diet and lifestyle. Are you eating enough fresh fruits, vegetables, and whole grains? Are you getting adequate fluids in your diet? Are you getting enough exercise? If you can answer yes to those questions and are still having difficulty with elimination, try using a bulk-forming digestive aid such as psyllium or flaxseed before resorting to a stimulant laxative. If you have experienced a significant change in your bowel habits for no obvious reason, discuss your situation with your health-care adviser before embarking on a course of laxatives.

HOW TO USE SENNA

Most senna preparations are standardized to contain a predictable quantity of sennosides. In Sennokot, each tablet delivers 8.6 milligrams of sennosides, with the usual dosage ranging from two to four tablets at a time. Other preparations usually provide a specific amount of dried senna leaves or pods, ranging from 150 to 450 milligrams. Standard doses are more difficult to get in herbal teas containing senna. If you prefer to use a tea, become familiar with a specific brand, and steep it a consistent amount of time to ensure a reproducible response.

AYURVEDA AND SENNA

Senna is considered a laxative of moderate potency. With its bitter and cooling effects on the physiology, it is pacifying to Pitta and Kapha. Used excessively, it can be depleting and aggravating to Vata. According to Ayurveda, the digestive tract should be prepared before taking senna by eating lightly and increasing your intake of oily foods such as sesame seeds or ghee (clarified butter). This "oleation" is said to ensure a smoother, more comfortable elimination in response to the herbal laxative.

PRECAUTIONS

Although occasionally taking an herbal laxative is generally safe, there are risks associated with regular usage. Radiologists have described a pattern on colon X-rays associated with long-term laxative use called "cathartic colon." A recent report showed that this pattern, which consists of dilated portions of the large intestines and loss of the usual anatomic complexity, is occasionally seen in people who chronically use senna, and may reflect damage to the colon and its nerve input.[17]

The possible role of senna use in development of colon cancer has been studied for many years, and the general consensus is that there is not an increased risk of cancer, even in chronic users of herbal laxatives.[18] A benign condition that has been associated with senna is called melanosis coli.[19] This describes a dark staining of the lining of the colon that can be seen on internal colonoscopic examination. Senna stimulates the accumulation of pigment in the colon, which usually becomes apparent within a year of regular laxative use. If senna is discontinued, the pigmentation gradually fades over the course of about a year. Although this condition has been known for over thirty years, it has not been associated with any clinical problems.

Senna is usually considered to be among the safer laxatives in women who are breastfeeding, for only a small portion is absorbed and enters the bloodstream.[20] Studies have shown that metabolic products of senna do enter the breast milk but at levels of about one one-thousandth those of the mother.[21] The occasional use of senna probably causes no measurable harm to the infant, but should raise the question of what more can be done to normalize digestive function through appropriate diet and lifestyle choices.

Circulatory/Respiratory	Detoxifier	Digestive	Immune Enhancer	Men's Health
	X	X		
Metabolic	Nervine	Rejuvenative	Rheumatic	Women's Health

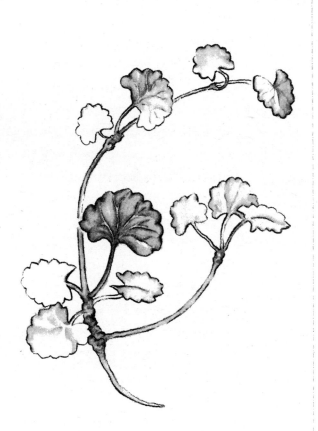

CENTELLA ASIATICA

FAMILIAR: **gotu kola**
LATIN: *Centella asiatica*
SANSKRIT: brahmi

Gotu kola, also known as Indian pennywort, carries two different Latin names, *Centella asiatica* and *Hydrocotyle asiatica,* both referring to the same plant. Its name in Sanskrit, *brahmi,* means consciousness or wisdom. In India several different botanical specimens have been named brahmi, for their influence on improving memory and clarifying thinking. The most widely available form of brahmi, gotu kola is one of the most important plants in Ayurveda. It is used for a wide spectrum of illnesses ranging from indigestion to dementia. Native to India, it can now be found throughout the world including the southern United States.

Described in the original Ayurvedic textbooks several thousand years ago, gotu kola was also known to Chinese physicians for its ability to promote longevity. It carries a long-standing reputation as a wound healer and brain enhancer. Gotu kola has gained a recent following in the West among students, who believe it can improve their ability to retain information while preparing for examinations.

Although gotu kola has a long history of enhancing cognitive function, it has thus far received scarce scientific attention in this area.

BOTANICAL AND PHYTOCHEMICAL INFORMATION

Gotu kola is a perennial creeping plant with distinctive leaves that look like open Japanese fans. It grows throughout India, preferring marshlands, where it has ready access to fresh water. The trailing herb bears small white flowers and lays down roots along its stems. The leaves, which can be eaten fresh, are harvested throughout the year. Dried aerial parts are used internally and as an external poultice.

Gotu kola is a chemically complex herb that contains many different components including alkaloids, glycosides, sterols, and tannins. Unique substances identified as brahmoside and brahminoside may account for its calming effect. Other chemical constituents in gotu kola have antibiotic and wound-healing properties.

THE SCIENCE OF GOTU KOLA

Although gotu kola is best known in India as a mind tonic, most research has centered on its ability to facilitate the healing of wounds. Creams and ointments containing gotu kola extract have been shown to hasten wound healing and improved the strength of the scar that forms.[1] A component of gotu kola increases the synthesis of collagen, enabling wounds to heal faster and better. Taking advantage of these qualities, gotu kola has been used to help heal skin ulcers, traumatic injuries, and surgical wounds.

Taken internally, gotu kola has been shown effective in reducing leg edema in people with chronic venous insufficiency.[2] It reduces pain, cramping, and swelling without any serious side effects. It may also provide some value in shrinking varicose veins.

Gotu kola's value in a number of other health concerns is just beginning to be explored scientifically. Reports have suggested that it may be helpful in herpes infections, cancer, and stomach ulcers, but more research is needed. Despite its accepted role in Ayurveda as an herb to enhance mental function, the only scientific study to look at this issue was performed over thirty years ago in mentally disabled children.[3] Researchers reported that those who took gotu kola for twelve weeks had better attention and concentration ability. Further studies are clearly indicated on this potentially important property.

Another herb that has traditionally been called brahmi has the Latin name *Bacopa monniera*. It has recently become available in the West, with reports indicating that it influences brain neurotransmitter levels and has potent antioxidant activity.[4] These effects may help explain its common usage in India to improve memory and treat insomnia and anxiety. An animal study has shown that brahmi significantly enhances both memory and performance.[5]

THE PRACTICAL USE OF GOTU KOLA

Gotu kola is valued for its purifying and balancing influence. We recommend gotu kola when people are having difficulty concentrating because of mental turbulence. The combination of a meditation practice and gotu kola can effectively reduce anxiety and improve mental clarity. It combines well with chamomile or valerian for a gentle sleep aid.

Gotu kola tea is prescribed for headaches, particularly when a person is detoxifying from alcohol or caffeine. We often prescribe gotu kola as a general rejuvenative herb for people recovering from illness or surgery. Herbalized brahmi oil is applied to the skin to soothe irritations and is taken as nose drops to calm an agitated mind.

HOW TO USE GOTU KOLA

As a tea, steep one teaspoon of dried gotu kola leaves in a cup of boiling water. Sweetened with honey, it can be sipped before bed to induce a deep, restful sleep.

A cup of tea can also be helpful in relieving headache or indigestion from overeating or a poor diet.

As a paste for skin conditions, combine one-quarter cup of dried gotu kola leaves with one-quarter cup of chamomile, and steep in one-half cup of boiling water for ten minutes. Strain and blend the liquid with cornstarch to make a thick paste. Apply lightly for relief of irritated skin. Rinse off the paste with room-temperature water once it has dried. As an oil for itchy and irritated skin, boil one-half cup of dried brahmi leaves in two cups of water until the volume is reduced by half. Remove the leaves and add one cup of almond or sesame oil and slowly boil off the water until you are left with the herbalized oil. This can be used for local skin or muscular concerns as well as for a general massage. Dried gotu kola is usually available in one-third- to one-half-gram tablets or capsules. The standard dose is 1 to 2 grams daily to improve memory.

AYURVEDA AND GOTU KOLA

Brahmi has many uses in Ayurveda. In addition to its role in memory, it is commonly prescribed to reduce fever, treat eczema, and relieve respiratory congestion. It has a mild laxative and diuretic effect, and plays a traditional role as a blood purifier. Taking advantage of its wound-healing properties, women are encouraged to soak in brahmi sitz baths after giving birth, to soothe irritated tissues.

Gotu kola is bitter, pungent, and sweet in taste, and cooling to the body. It can be useful in balancing all three doshas, but is particularly effective for Pitta-aggravated nervous systems.

PRECAUTIONS

Care must be taken when applying gotu kola topically, as it can occasionally cause an allergic dermatitis. In very high doses it may aggravate rather than relieve headaches.

Circulatory/Respiratory	Detoxifier	Digestive	Immune Enhancer	Men's Health
	X			
Metabolic	Nervine	Rejuvenative	Rheumatic	Women's Health
	X	X		

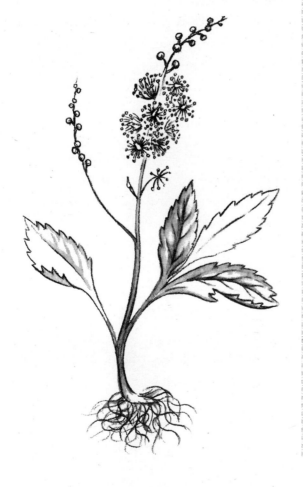

CIMICIFUGA RACEMOSA

FAMILIAR: **black cohosh**
LATIN: *Cimicifuga racemosa*

Black cohosh is a traditional Native American herb that has been employed in the treatment of women's health issues for thousands of years. It was called squawroot by North American Indians for its reputation in easing the pains of childbirth. Although originally a component of the American pharmacopoeia, black cohosh fell out of favor in the 1930s when a paper disputed its efficacy.[1] Despite its abandonment by American medical doctors, black cohosh has been accepted by European physicians for the past half-century. Over one and a half million German women have safely used black cohosh, and the German Commission E has approved it for the treatment of menstrual complaints and menopausal symptoms. After being ignored for over sixty years, black cohosh is again gaining in popularity in the United States.

BOTANICAL AND PHYTOCHEMICAL INFORMATION

Black cohosh, native to the eastern half of North America, can be found from Canada to Florida. It has elongated, serrated leaves and produces spires with clusters of tiny white flowers. The roots are harvested in the fall from this perennial shrub that grows to about six feet in height. Black cohosh is now widely cultivated in Europe, where its roots are collected and dried.

Black cohosh contains a number of glycosides, flavonoids, and terpenes. It also contains tannins and salycilates. Although the active constituents have not been fully characterized, the most popular proprietary form of black cohosh, known as Remifemin, is standardized to contain two milligrams of a chemical, 27-deoxyacetein. Some studies have suggested that black cohosh has estrogenic effects, but the chemicals responsible for its hormonal properties still need to be identified.

THE SCIENCE OF BLACK COHOSH

Several studies over the past forty years have evaluated the effects of black cohosh on menopausal symptoms. A German study evaluated the benefits of black cohosh in over six hundred menopausal women and reported that almost 80 percent noticed some type of improvement in their symptoms, with very rare side effects.[2] Other studies have found that black cohosh improves both the physical and psychological symptoms of women going through menopause as soon as one month after starting the herb.[3, 4] A German study in eighty women found that those taking black cohosh had less anxiety, fewer hot flashes, and improved vaginal tissue.[5] When compared with a standard estrogen replacement drug, those taking black cohosh reported better relief of menopausal symptoms without substantial side effects. Another German report found that over 40 percent of women taking hormone replacement for the treatment of hot flashes were able to reduce or eliminate their medication.[6]

The question of how black cohosh relieves menopausal symptoms has not yet been answered. It has been suggested that it acts as a phytoestrogen, and in some studies components have been shown to bind to estrogen receptors and influence the release of pituitary hormones.[7] Other reports, however, have not been able to show a definite estrogen-like effect on the uterus.[8] How black cohosh works to decrease the hot flashes and psychological symptoms of menopause is not just an academic question, for if it does act as a natural estrogen, it is important to determine the optimal dose, how long it should be taken, and if there are any long-term side effects.

Does black cohosh have any role in the prevention of osteoporosis or heart disease? Although one study in animals suggested that black cohosh could improve bone density, this property has not been evaluated in women.[9] From a scientific perspective, we know that black cohosh improves the short-term physical and mental symptoms of menopause, but we do not know its long-term effects. Most reports emphasize black cohosh's safety, particularly in comparison with standard hormone replacement therapy.[10]

Although black cohosh has other traditional uses, including treatment for premenstrual syndrome, arthritis, and high blood pressure, the scientific basis of these claims is limited. A study from the 1960s suggested that black cohosh could dilate blood vessels and lower blood pressure, but there has not been recent confirmation of this effect.[11] Other reports have listed both anti-inflammatory and blood-sugar-lowering properties of black cohosh, but the clinical application of those laboratory findings remains to be explored.[12, 13]

THE PRACTICAL USE OF BLACK COHOSH

Black cohosh is effective in treating the hot flashes associated with menopause. It may also have some value in dampening the emotional ups and downs that are often associated with the physiological changes of midlife. At this time we do not know if black cohosh provides protection against osteoporosis or heart disease. If you are taking black cohosh in lieu of estrogen replacement, be certain to get enough calcium in your diet (1,500 milligrams per day) and perform regular weight-bearing and aerobic exercise.

Traditionally, black cohosh has been useful in the treatment of a wide range of women's health concerns. It may help to reduce the congestion, breast tenderness, and irritability associated with the hormonal changes preceding menstruation. Believed capable of reducing menstrual cramping, black cohosh was also recommended during childbirth, where it was used to regulate uterine contractions. Although this property has not been scientifically verified, black cohosh should be avoided during pregnancy because of its potential stimulatory effects on the uterus.

In addition to its role in women's health, black cohosh has been promoted for the treatment of joint and muscle pain. Native American healers have used black cohosh for its anti-inflammatory effects, possibly a result of its aspirin-like salicylate compounds. Black cohosh has also been traditionally employed in the treatment of asthma, where its relaxant properties are believed to reduce airway restriction. These many traditional healing properties of black cohosh are clearly worthy of further scientific exploration.

HOW TO USE BLACK COHOSH

Black cohosh is readily available in health-food stores, in tablets and extracts. Most American herbal companies are following the lead of European brands, offering tablets standardized to contain 2.5 percent tripertene glycosides. As noted above, the most popular form of black cohosh in Europe, Remifemin, contains a standard 2 milligrams of 27-deoxyacetein. Extracts of black cohosh are also increasingly available. The usual dose is two tablets or forty drops of a standardized liquid extract twice daily. Some formulas combine black cohosh with St. John's wort to provide greater mood-stabilizing benefit.

AYURVEDA AND BLACK COHOSH

The ancient Ayurvedic physicians did not know black cohosh, but it can be analyzed according to Ayurvedic principles. It carries the bitter and pungent tastes, and has a cooling influence on the physiology. It can balance both Pitta and Kapha, and may aggravate Vata after prolonged use.

PRECAUTIONS

Black cohosh has a long history of safety. The German Commission E suggests it may cause occasional stomach discomfort and does not recommend its use for longer than six months. Black cohosh is not to be taken during pregnancy.

Circulatory/Respiratory	Detoxifier	Digestive	Immune Enhancer	Men's Health

Metabolic	Nervine	Rejuvenative	Rheumatic	Women's Health
			X	X

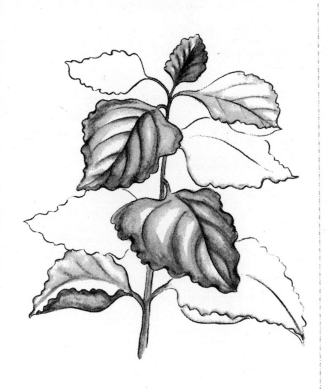

COLEUS
FORSKOHLII

FAMILIAR: **forskolin, coleus**
LATIN: *Coleus forskohlii*
SANSKRIT: pashanbhedi, balaka

Members of the coleus species are familiar as popular colorful houseplants, but the little-known perennial *Coleus forskohlii* made pharmacological history when it was discovered to have unique medicinal properties. Native to the subtropical zones of India, Nepal, and Thailand, coleus has a long traditional history of benefit in the treatment of respiratory problems, heart ailments, and skin conditions. In the early 1970s we learned that many of the therapeutic effects of coleus result from its content of a unique substance, forskolin. This chemical increases the cellular levels of cyclic AMP (cAMP), one of the most elementary compounds of life. This compound is intricately involved in our most basic biological functions, from the regulation of blood pressure to the response of the immune system. Since its discovery, over twelve thousand scientific articles have appeared, investigating the effects of forskolin on cellular physiology. This member of the mint family is demonstrating potentially far-reaching clinical applications.

BOTANICAL AND PHYTOCHEMICAL INFORMATION

The *Coleus forskohlii* plant grows on temperate mountain slopes between one thousand and six thousand feet. The small shrub grows to about two feet in height, with new plants easily propagated by stem cuttings. The paired alternate fragrant leaves are commonly cultivated as a pickling spice in the Gujarat district of India. Flowers, leaves, and stems all contain forskolin, with the tuberous roots and stem base containing the highest concentrations.[1]

A number of diterpenoids have been identified in coleus, of which forskolin has received the most attention. Forskolin activates the enzyme adenylate cyclase, which increases the formation of cAMP.[2] Increased concentrations of cAMP within cells leads to the relaxation of smooth muscles, and diminishes allergic and inflammatory responses.[3, 4] All the clinical effects of coleus cannot be fully accounted for by changes in cAMP or the chemical forskolin, but the other important active plant constituents have not yet been identified.

THE SCIENCE OF COLEUS

Forskolin has been most studied in the treatment of cardiovascular diseases and asthma. Animal studies have shown that forskolin can improve the efficiency of heart muscle contractions and lower blood pressure by relaxing the muscles that control blood vessel tone.[5] These effects have been shown to be clinically beneficial in patients with cardiac failure, whose hearts responded to intravenous forskolin by pumping more strongly without consuming more energy.[6] Forskolin's ability to inhibit the tendency of platelets to clump together could provide additional benefit in reducing coronary blood vessel blockages.[7] The importance of these findings in the prevention and treatment of heart dis-

ease remains to be fully explored through further research.

Forskolin has also been shown to reduce the tendency for the respiratory passages to go into spasm, making it a potentially useful remedy for asthma. Animal studies have shown forskolin to reduce the allergic response to substances that trigger the closing of small airways in the lungs.[8, 9] The applicability of these findings to people has been supported in studies that have compared forskolin extract to standard asthma pharmaceuticals. Inhaled doses of forskolin in asthmatic patients improved their breathing function without the usual jittery side effects associated with asthma medications.[10–12] The improvement seemed to result from relaxation of the smooth muscles that regulate the size of the airways. The question that still needs to be answered is whether coleus taken orally has as substantial a benefit as inhaled forskolin in patients with reactive airway disease.

Forskolin has been tested in other conditions with promising but, at times, mixed results. Animal studies have shown that forskolin eye drops reduce the pressure in the eyes, suggesting that it may have a role in the treatment of glaucoma.[13] This action has been tested in people, with some reports showing a benefit and others not.[14–16] Taking advantage of its ability to dilate blood vessels, researchers have tested forskolin in the treatment of male impotence and found it potentially useful in both animals and humans without significant side effects.[17]

Preliminary studies have suggested that forskolin may also have antidepressant and cancer fighting properties.[18, 19]

The diverse potentially therapeutic effects of forskolin reflect its ability to influence one of the most basic biochemicals of life, cyclic AMP. The traditional healers of India and Nepal recognized forskolin's value in disorders of circulation, breathing, and digestion. Medical science is just beginning to explore the full range of therapeutic applications of this unassuming member of the mint family.

THE PRACTICAL USE OF FORSKOLIN

Most people will not have access to pharmaceutically pure forskolin that can be inhaled, injected, or applied to the eyes. Standardized powdered extracts for oral consumption are increasingly available, derived from the dried leaves or roots of the *Coleus forskohlii* plant. The traditional use of *Coleus forskohlii* for respiratory and circulatory disorders usually involved ingesting a strong infusion of ground roots and leaves several times per day. A paste of the powdered herb applied directly to the skin has also been used for eczema and infections.

Before ingesting forskolin for its lung or circulatory effects, discuss its use with a health-care provider who is familiar with this herb and can closely monitor your response. Do not mix forskolin with prescribed medications.

HOW TO USE FORSKOLIN

Coleus forskohlii products available in the West are usually standardized to contain between 0.25 percent and 1 percent forskolin. Tablets provide between 1 and 5 milligrams per dose. The usual recommended daily intake is 3 to 15 milligrams in three divided doses. The effects of forskolin are rapid and short-acting, so, if you are taking it for a specific health concern, such as mild asthma or elevated blood pressure, you will know within a week whether or not it is providing benefit for your condition.

AYURVEDA AND FORSKOLIN

The predominant taste of forskolin is bitter, with a secondary weak astringency. It has a cooling effect on the physiology. This herb is pacifying to Pitta and Kapha. It can be mildly aggravating to Vata if used for a prolonged time.

PRECAUTIONS

No serious adverse reactions have been reported with forskolin, and animal studies have suggested that it is well tolerated. Since studies evaluating interactions with pharmaceutical agents have not been performed, we do not advise mixing forskolin with asthma or blood pressure medica- tions unless you are under the supervision of a knowledgeable health-care adviser.

Circulatory/Respiratory	Detoxifier	Digestive	Immune Enhancer	Men's Health
X				
Metabolic	Nervine	Rejuvenative	Rheumatic	Women's Health

COMMIPHORA MUKUL

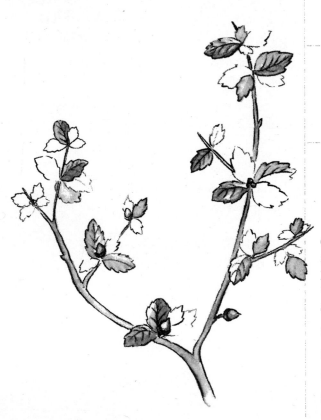

FAMILIAR: **guggulu, gum gugal**
LATIN: *Commiphora mukul*
SANSKRIT: Guggulu

Guggulu is one of Ayurveda's most important purifying herbs. It cleanses unhealthy tissues, increases the white blood cell count, and rejuvenates the skin. Traditionally it has been considered the consummate blood detoxifier, useful in any condition characterized by congestion or stagnation. Derived from the resin of a small tree native to India, guggulu is a close relative of myrrh, one of the gifts offered to the baby Jesus by the Three Wise Men.

Guggulu was well known to the Ayurvedic sages Charaka and Sushruta. In the original texts from over two thousand years ago, guggulu was recommended to clear the sinuses of congestion, relieve chronic skin disorders, treat obesity, shrink swollen glands, and cool inflamed joints. It is fascinating how medical science is now validating many of the traditional uses for this ancient herbal medicine.

BOTANICAL AND PHYTOCHEMICAL INFORMATION

The guggulu tree grows to about ten feet high in both northern and southern India as well as regions of the Middle East. The medicinal substance is a yellowish resin exuded when the inner bark of the tree is injured. The resin is usually harvested in the winter from branches that have dropped their leaves.

The resin obtained from guggulu trees contains several different chemical compounds that can be extracted with organic solvents. These soluble portions have documented anti-inflammatory and cholesterol-lowering properties. Most current herbal formulas of guggulu contain standardized amounts of the cholesterol-lowering constituents, known as guggulsterones. Most studies on guggulu have used a 2.5 percent extract of guggulsterones standardized to a 50-milligram dose. This extract is commonly referred to as gugulipid. Other important components of guggulu, including organic acids and sterols, seem to possess anti-inflammatory activity.

THE SCIENCE OF GUGGULU

Scientific research has focused on two main properties of guggulu: its ability to lower serum cholesterol levels and its anti-inflammatory effect. Sushruta extolled guggulu's penetrating properties, used to dissolve the deposition of ama (toxins) in the channels of circulation. The development of atherosclerosis, known as *medoroga* in Ayurveda, encompassed much of our modern understanding of this illness. According to Ayurveda, eating excessively rich foods and not getting enough exercise leads to an accumulation of fat in the blood that eventually builds up and obstructs the *srotas,* or channels of circulation. Guggulu helps to prevent and reverse this process by stimulating digestion and clearing fat from the blood.

Studies dating back to the late 1960s suggested that taking guggulu could result in significant reductions in blood levels of cholesterol and triglycerides.[1] More-recent reports have confirmed these preliminary findings in both animals and people. Researchers in India found that men taking 50 milligrams of gugulipid twice a day for six months had about a 12-percent drop in their cholesterol levels.[2] Side effects in a few patients included mild headache, nausea, and stomach gas, but over 95 percent of subjects took the herb regularly without difficulty.

In another study, gugulipid was compared to a standard cholesterol-lowering drug, clofibrate, in over two hundred patients with raised cholesterol or triglyceride levels. Gugulipid was more effective than clofibrate in patients with high cholesterol, slightly less effective in patients with high triglycerides, and equivalent in people with elevations in both. Perhaps most important, patients taking gugulipid had elevations in their HDL cholesterol levels, the so-called good cholesterol component.[3]

In addition to its cholesterol-lowering activity, guggulu reduces the stickiness of platelets,[4] the blood components that stop us from bleeding when we cut ourselves, but that also contribute to undesired clotting of blood vessels. The combination of guggulu's fat-lowering properties and its ability to slightly thin the blood makes it a desirable substance to reduce the risk of heart disease and stroke.

Guggulu's other important medicinal effect is its ability to reduce inflammation. It holds an established place in the Ayurvedic pharmacy as a first-line treatment for arthritis. Animal studies comparing guggulu to established anti-inflammatory medicines such as ibuprofen and phenylbutazone showed that guggulu was equally effective in reducing joint swelling.[5] The anti-inflammatory benefit of guggulu has also been found useful in the treatment of acne. In a study comparing guggulu to the antibiotic tetracycline, guggulu was slightly more effective, particularly in people with oily skin.[6]

THE PRACTICAL USE OF GUGGULU

Traditionally, many therapeutic properties are attributed to guggulu. It has been used for thousands of years in the treatment of obesity, where it is believed to stimulate the digestion of stored toxins. It can be applied directly to festering skin sores, including acne lesions. As a mouthwash, guggulu can be helpful in the treatment of canker sores and gingivitis. Wherever there is a condition of stagnation, guggulu's penetrating properties can clear away the toxins.

We use guggulu liberally at the Chopra Center in people who have accumulated toxicity from significant life stresses. People who are recovering from serious illnesses, who have required prolonged courses of antibiotics, or who have recently stopped using recreational drugs or alcohol benefit from guggulu's detoxifying properties.

In people with elevated cholesterol levels, guggulu can be an initial approach before resorting to the more potent cholesterol-lowering drugs. Although it is traditionally used in the treatment of rheumatoid arthritis, we have found guggulu to be most helpful in relieving the discomfort of people with nonspecific pain. Myofascial pain syndrome, fibromyalgia, and rheumatism are conditions that often respond to the cleansing activity of guggulu.

A combination of guggulu and Triphala is helpful in strengthening digestive power. The mixture is particularly beneficial when someone has both weak digestion and irregular elimination. We use a suspension of guggulu as a gargle for sore throats, mouth sores, and gingivitis. A crushed tablet mixed with warm water is swished in the mouth or gargled several times daily until the soreness resolves.

HOW TO USE GUGGULU

Guggulu is now readily available through several herbal producers. Since most studies have found that 25 milligrams of guggulsterones three times daily is effective in reducing elevated cholesterol levels, be certain that you are receiving this amount. Some formulations list the total guggulu content, which should be at least 500 milligrams per tablet. For the treatment of rheumatic conditions, try taking two tablets three times a day after meals. You should see a response within two weeks.

As a gargle or mouthwash, crush a tablet in one-half cup of warm water and use three times daily. This same mixture can be applied to superficial skin wounds to facilitate healing.

AYURVEDA AND GUGGULU

As one of Ayurveda's primary detoxifying substances, guggulu is beneficial in a wide range of conditions. A complex herb, carrying four of the six tastes—bitter, pungent, astringent, and sweet—it is especially effective for stabilizing Vata and Kapha imbalances without irritating Pitta. Whenever there is an accumulation of toxicity in the system, guggulu can be a powerful aid to digesting and eliminating it.

PRECAUTIONS

Guggulu is slightly heating and is occasionally associated with mild digestive discomfort. In view of its role in reducing platelet stickiness, it should not be used in patients receiving blood-thinning medications.

Circulatory/Respiratory	Detoxifier	Digestive	Immune Enhancer	Men's Health
X	X			
Metabolic	Nervine	Rejuvenative	Rheumatic	Women's Health
X			X	

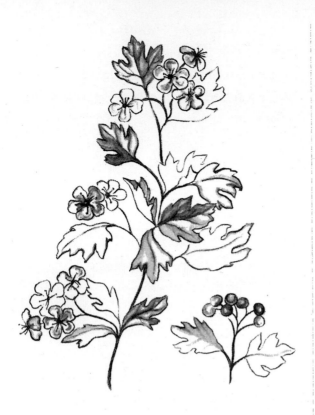

CRATAEGUS
OXYACANTHA

FAMILIAR: **hawthorn, May blossom**
LATIN: *Crataegus oxyacantha*

Well known to European healers of medieval times, hawthorn was identified as a sacred herb, supposed to be the source of Christ's crown of thorns. During the fourteenth century, the unusual smell of hawthorn berries became associated with the bubonic plague, and for the next two hundred years it was avoided as a healing aid. By the 1600s, hawthorn regained its reputation as an important herbal rejuvenative through the writings of the famous English herbalist Nicholas Culpeper. Traditionally used as a treatment for urinary tract problems, it came to be known by Western herbalists as an important cardiac tonic. Modern scientific studies have confirmed the circulatory benefits of the bright red berries and flowering tops of this familiar tree, now found throughout the temperate zones of Europe, North America, and Asia.

BOTANICAL AND PHYTOCHEMICAL INFORMATION

A member of the rose family, the deciduous hawthorn tree, with its sharp thorns, can grow to heights of thirty feet. It blooms in small white flowers with roselike petals during the spring, accounting for one of hawthorn's common names, May blossom. The flowers give rise to small red berries with one or two seeds. The dried berries have traditionally been the source of the herbal medicine, although active phytochemicals have also been identified in the flowers and leaves.

A wide range of chemical constituents is present in hawthorn, including polysaccharides, amines, tannins, phytosterols, and organic acids. Most scientific attention has focused on hawthorn's flavonoid components, particularly quercetin, rutin, and the proanthocyanidins, also known as procyanidins. Also abundant in grape seeds, pine bark, cranberries, beans, and bran, proanthocyanidins have potent antioxidant properties and protective effects on collagen tissue. According to some reports, proanthocyanidins are more potent neutralizers of free radicals than the antioxidant vitamins C and E.[1] The proanthocyanidins identified in hawthorn include catechin and epicatechin, also present in green tea and red wine. These and other natural chemicals in hawthorn contribute to its beneficial effects on cardiovascular health.

THE SCIENCE OF HAWTHORN

There are several possible ways in which hawthorn may contribute to cardiac health. It has a mild blood-pressure-lowering effect, believed due to its ability to block the enzyme that activates the chemical, angiotensin, a substance that constricts blood vessels and induces the kidney to retain salt.[2] Many modern blood pressure medicines act by blocking this angiotensin-converting enzyme (ACE); these are known as ACE inhibitors.

Hawthorn has also been found effective in lowering blood cholesterol levels and strengthening the collagen component of connective tissues.[3, 4] These combined effects can slow the development of athero-sclerosis in heart blood vessels that leads to heart attacks. Some of the most interesting studies on hawthorn have found that it can reduce the damage sustained by heart tissue as a result of blocked coronary arteries.[5, 6] These heart-protecting effects of hawthorn are mainly due to the free radical–neutralizing properties of the abundant proanthocyanidins it contains.[7] Hawthorn may also help dilate coronary blood vessels, allowing for greater oxygen and energy delivery to the heart.[8] In addition to limiting the amount of heart muscle that is injured, hawthorn reduces the risk of serious heart rhythm irregularities triggered by inadequate blood flow.[9]

A number of reports from Europe have shown that the diverse effects of hawthorn on the circulatory system can be of benefit to people with heart disease. In one study of seventy-eight patients with chronic heart failure, those taking a daily dose of hawthorn extract had a lowering of their blood pressure, a reduction in their heart rate, and a significant improvement in their exercise tolerance.[10] Another report, from Germany, evaluated 136 people with heart failure and found that both objective and subjective measurements of cardiac function improved.[11] Measurements of cardiac function improved, and people reported a better quality of life.

Hawthorn is generally very well tolerated by heart patients without serious side effects. Considering its low toxicity and many positive actions, it is clearly worthy of further scientific research to clarify its rightful place in the treatment of heart disease, the most pressing health concern of our age.

THE PRACTICAL USE OF HAWTHORN

In European countries, hawthorn is often prescribed by physicians in the treatment of mild heart conditions, characterized by nonspecific fatigue, exercise intolerance, and occasional palpitations. It is best viewed as a tonic that must be taken daily for several weeks before a noticeable benefit is seen. Hawthorn may have a mild sedative effect, adding to its value in stress-exacerbated conditions.

If you have a diagnosed heart condition, be certain to discuss the use of hawthorn with your health-care provider before using it. Do not abruptly discontinue any of your current heart medicines without the approval of, and close monitoring by, your doctor.

HOW TO USE HAWTHORN

Hawthorn is widely available in a variety of preparations, including tablets of dried berries, tinctures, and flower extracts. Dried-berry tablets or capsules containing approximately 500 milligrams are the most common forms obtainable in the United States. Extracts standardized to contain 1 to 3 percent vitexin, one of the isolated flavonoids in hawthorn, are also available. The usual dose is .5 gram to 1 gram of the dried berries twice daily.

In Germany, most hawthorn is in the form of a water-ethanol extract of the leaves and flowers. The dose recommended by the German Commission E is 160 to 900 milligrams per day, corresponding to 3.5 to 20 milligrams of flavonoids. Standardized extracts available here usually contain about 1.8 milligrams of flavonoids, so two to four tablets daily will provide a dosage within the suggested range.

AYURVEDA AND HAWTHORN

Although not recognized in the ancient Ayurvedic formularies, hawthorn's effects on the doshas can be understood by looking at its basic properties. The predominant tastes of hawthorn berries are sour, bitter, and sweet. It has a mildly heating potency on the physiology. Hawthorn is pacifying to Vata and neutral to Pitta, but may be aggravating to Kapha in high dosages.

PRECAUTIONS

Hawthorn is a generally safe herbal nutritional substance. Studies from the early 1980s reported very low toxicity in animals.[12] Despite the fact that hawthorn is well tolerated, it should be used cautiously by people with heart ailments. Studies assessing its interactions with standard cardiac drugs have not been performed. It is generally not recommended for women who are pregnant or breastfeeding.

Circulatory/Respiratory	Detoxifier	Digestive	Immune Enhancer	Men's Health
X				
Metabolic	Nervine	Rejuvenative	Rheumatic	Women's Health

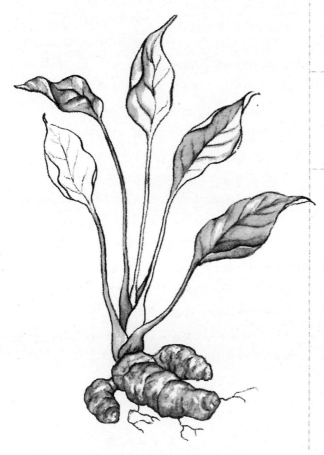

CURCURMA LONGA

FAMILIAR: **turmeric**
LATIN: *Curcurma longa*
SANSKRIT: haridra

This beautiful yellow spice belongs to the same family as ginger. Known primarily as a culinary herb in the West, turmeric holds an established position in healing systems around the world, including India, China, and the Polynesian islands. It is a component of most curry powder blends and contributes to the yellow color of many mustard preparations. Used as a cosmetic agent in ancient India, it was known to heal the skin as well as provide a lustrous golden glow.

BOTANICAL AND PHYTOCHEMICAL INFORMATION

Culinary and medicinal turmeric is derived from the rhizomes of this perennial herb that grows to about three feet high. The usable part is harvested in the winter, boiled or steamed, and then dried. Although about 5 percent of the rhizome is composed of an essential oil, most turmeric is available as a powder.

Chemicals identified in turmeric include curcumin, tumerone, and zingiberone, along with a carotene equivalent to 50 IU of vitamin A per 100 grams. The medicinal effects of turmeric are probably related to the curcumin, which has been shown to have potent antioxidant properties.[1]

THE SCIENCE OF TURMERIC

Turmeric is a pharmacy unto itself. A wealth of scientific studies have demonstrated that this golden spice can have health-promoting effects on the digestive, cardiovascular, rheumatic, and immune systems. It has a very high safety profile without serious side effects at usual dosages.

Turmeric has a soothing effect on the digestive system, with studies showing that it helps to increase the mucous protective lining of the stomach, reducing the risk of ulcers due to stress or drugs.[2] It has a protective effect on the liver and can help reduce elevated blood cholesterol levels.[3, 4]

The most common medicinal uses of turmeric involve its anti-inflammatory properties. Constituents of turmeric have been shown to suppress inflammation by blocking the production of certain prostaglandin chemicals.[5] Through a similar mechanism, it has been shown to keep platelets from sticking together, which, along with its documented cholesterol-lowering effect and its ability to suppress the growth of blood vessel muscle cells, may give turmeric an important role in lowering the risk of heart attacks.[6]

One of turmeric's traditional uses has been in the treatment of arthritis, and scientific studies have suggested that, alone or in combination with other herbs, it can reduce pain and stiffness.[7, 8] Several studies in animals have demonstrated that turmeric can prevent or inhibit the development of certain cancer cells, but whether this is relevant to people has yet to be determined.[9, 10] It does seem to help the body detoxify itself of potentially cancer-causing substances.[11]

Turmeric has long been used as a natural antibiotic agent. Studies from around the world have confirmed that components of this multitalented spice can inhibit the growth of bacteria, yeast, and viruses.[12, 13]

The German Commission E has determined that turmeric is effective in digestive disturbances, with the particular effect of stimulating the gallbladder to empty. It is not recommended for use in people with known gallstones.

PRACTICAL USES FOR TURMERIC

Turmeric powder adds its pleasant taste and beautiful color to soups and sautéed vegetable dishes, and can be used liberally as a culinary spice. Its traditional purifying effect makes it a useful spice for people participating in a detoxification program. Turmeric can be taken at the earliest sign of a sore throat or cough by sprinkling it onto organic honey and licking a teaspoon every two hours. It can also be added to a variety of herbal teas, including blends of chamomile, licorice, and slippery elm when facing a cold or flu. Occasionally, capsules of turmeric are prescribed for the treatment of mild arthritic conditions. In patients facing cancer, we recommend the liberal use of turmeric in food dishes. It is also encouraged for people diagnosed with mild adult-onset diabetes mellitus.

Powdered turmeric mixed into a paste with water can be directly applied to pimples and other irritated skin lesions before bedtime. The bright yellow color may make you reluctant to use turmeric on your face during the day. Once the paste dries, the residual powder can be washed off with plain water.

HOW TO USE TURMERIC

Turmeric is widely available in grocery and Indian spice stores. It is a traditional component of most curry spice blends in which it combines well with cumin, coriander, and fenugreek. A quarter teaspoon of turmeric added while cooking a cup of basmati rice adds its subtle flavor and golden color to the dish.

As a tea, add one-half teaspoon to a cup of boiling water, reduce the heat, and steep for ten minutes. Add a little honey and drink several times per day for a nagging cold or flu. It combines well with fresh gingerroot and cardamom.

If you have a sore throat, scoop up three-quarters of a teaspoon of honey and add as much turmeric powder as will stick to the honey. Then slowly lick the honey-turmeric mixture, allowing it to coat your throat as you swallow it. This can be repeated many times per day until your throat discomfort subsides.

For skin eruptions, take one-half teaspoon of turmeric powder and add a few drops of water at a time until you have a thick paste. Then apply the mixture to an aggravated pimple and allow it to dry fully. Wash the caked powder off, and repeat up to four times daily. For irritated rashes on parts of your body other than your face, mix turmeric powder with ghee (clarified butter) or coconut oil, one-half teaspoon of turmeric per ounce of oil or ghee. Then massage the herbalized oil into the irritated area. Repeat this two or three times each day for several days. To benefit from turmeric's generalized inflammatory and detoxifying properties, take one teaspoon in low-fat milk three times daily.

AYURVEDA AND TURMERIC

Turmeric is an important cleansing and detoxifying agent in Ayurvedic medicine. Classified as bitter and mildly heating, it is used both internally and topically. For fevers, colds, and flu, turmeric can be added to coriander and cinnamon teas or taken mixed with honey. Mixing it with clarified butter or vegetable oil enhances its absorption. It can be applied directly to sites of irritated skin, in the form of a paste or ointment. Taken internally, it has a particular effect of balancing excessive Kapha.

PRECAUTIONS

Although no clinical problems have been reported, turmeric's effect on platelets theoretically suggests that high doses should be avoided by people on prescribed blood thinners.

Circulatory/Respiratory	Detoxifier	Digestive	Immune Enhancer	Men's Health
	X	X		
Metabolic	Nervine	Rejuvenative	Rheumatic	Women's Health
			X	

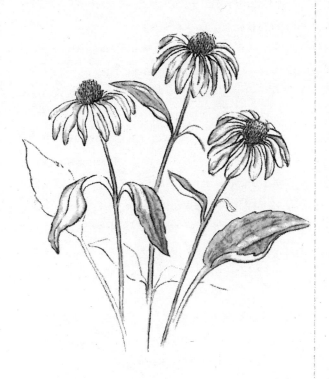

ECHINACEA
PURPUREA

FAMILIAR: **echinacea, purple coneflower**

LATIN: *Echinacea purpurea, Echinacea angustifolia, Echinacea pallida*

Perhaps the most popular herbal medicine in the United States, echinacea is native to North America. It was valued by Native Americans and prized by early European settlers. At least fourteen Native American tribes used echinacea medicinally for upper respiratory infections, snake bites, and toothaches. Of the nine known species of echinacea, three are commonly available today and seem to have equivalent actions. In addition to its reputed medicinal value, echinacea is popular in flower gardens for its attractive flowers.

Echinacea has been the subject of intense scientific investigations in both Europe and America to assess its reputation as an immune enhancer. Although not every study has yielded positive results, there is considerable evidence that echinacea can enhance our immunity. It is a generally safe herbal medicine with rare serious adverse effects reported despite millions of doses consumed annually.

BOTANICAL AND PHYTOCHEMICAL INFORMATION

Both the flowering tops and the roots of echinacea are used for medicinal purposes. All species of echinacea belong to the daisy family, and their flowers show characteristic raylike petals projecting from a central cone. The size of echinacea plants ranges from the smaller *E. angustifolia,* which is usually less than two feet in height, to the three-foot-tall *E. purpurea* to the even larger four-foot *E. pallida*. Echinacea's range extends from southern Canada through the central and eastern United States, with colors ranging from deep purple to light pink.

The chemical constituents of echinacea responsible for its medicinal properties have not been clearly characterized. Although sugars, glycosides, tannins, terpenes, and phenolic compounds have been identified, the polysaccharide component has received the most attention. Laboratory studies looking into echinacea have shown that a polysaccharide extract activates immune cells and inhibits the ability of bacteria to invade healthy cells. Several recent studies applying these test-tube findings to people have shown that the polysaccharide component of echinacea may be responsible for its anti-infective benefit in people.

THE SCIENCE OF ECHINACEA

Many studies have looked at the role of echinacea on the immune system. Studies in mice have shown that echinacea extract can enhance the production of immune-stimulating chemicals including interleukins and tumor necrosis factors, important in identifying and eliminating potentially harmful germs and cancer cells.[1] Components of echinacea also help attract and stimulate white blood cells, whose job it is to gobble up invading organisms.[2, 3] Known as macrophages, these warriors of the immune system are important in fighting viral, bacterial, and fungal infections. Interestingly, echinacea also contains natural anti-inflammatory chemicals, suggesting that this herb is intrinsically balanced so as not to overly excite an immune response.[4]

The ability of echinacea to influence immune function in people has been studied in both healthy volunteers and people with illnesses. In a recent review of five studies that measured immune function in healthy people taking echinacea, two showed a definite effect, while the other three did not.[5] The authors of this report pointed out that it was difficult to interpret the different results as the measurements of immune function, and the echinacea extract used was different in each study. In another report of twelve patients who had undergone surgery for cancerous tumors, echinacea did not have any detectable effect on their immune function.[6]

The important question regarding echinacea is whether or not it benefits people with real-life immune challenges. Although dozens of studies have looked at this question, most have weaknesses that make their reliable interpretation difficult.[7] Two well-designed investigations published in the early 1990s did find measurable benefit from the use of echinacea. In one, patients began taking echinacea drops at the start of a flu-like illness. Those who took a higher dose of echinacea extract had a faster recovery than people who took a lower dose or a placebo.[8] Another study, from Germany, looking at people with a tendency to get upper-respiratory infections found that those taking echinacea had fewer and less severe episodes over an eight-week period.[9]

Recent studies have been less clearcut. Subjects given daily doses of echinacea for twelve weeks showed no objective advantage in terms of a reduced frequency of respiratory infections, compared with those taking a placebo, although those on echinacea reported subjective benefits.[10] In yet another German study, people taking echinacea were followed for eight weeks and compared against those on a placebo. Although the average number of respiratory infections was .78 in the echinacea group and .93 in the placebo group, and the average length of a cold was 4.5 days in the echinacea group and 6.5 days in the placebo group, the differences did not reach statistical significance.[11] A more positive result was reported in a recent Swedish study in which people who took a concentrated echinacea extract at the start of a cold had faster relief of symptoms than those taking a placebo.[12]

Summarizing the findings of these various studies, it appears that echinacea has a benefit in reducing the symptoms of a cold or flu if it is taken early in the course. It is less certain that it has definite value as a preventive agent.

THE PRACTICAL USE OF ECHINACEA

Echinacea can provide natural support to your body's immune system for minor self-limiting respiratory infections. Keep some echinacea in your home pharmacy and begin taking it at the first signs of a cold or flu. Its role in other conditions where an immune boost may be valuable, such as other types of infections or cancer, has not been well documented. One report using echinacea in people with chronic fatigue syndrome and AIDS found that it could enhance immune function over the short term, but long-term follow-up was not available.[13] Whether you are basically healthy or are dealing with an illness that compromises your immune system, we do not recommend the use of echinacea on a regular basis, for it may lose its effectiveness after taking it steadily for a couple of weeks and not be helpful when you actually need it.

In addition to its internal use, echinacea has also had a traditional use as a topical medicinal substance. Dried herbal tablets can be crushed and suspended in water to be used as a gargle for sore throats. The juiced extract can also be applied directly to abrasions or sores to reduce the chance of infection.

HOW TO USE ECHINACEA

Echinacea is available in many forms today. Tablets and capsules containing the dried herb and tinctures are the most common products, although you can now find echinacea in teas, cold remedies, and even throat lozenges. Many herb manufacturers have standardized their doses to provide a specific percentage of chemical ingredients, usually 15 percent polysaccharides and 4 percent phenolic compounds. Tablets and capsules deliver between 125 and 300 milligrams of echinacea extract per dose. Recommended daily intake is between 500 milligrams and 1 gram in two or three divided doses.

Echinacea is also available as a liquid tincture, usually extracted in ethanol in a 1:1 or 1:2 dilution. The extracts can be derived solely from the root or may include material from seeds, leaves, and flowers. Echinacea extract is often combined with extracts of other herbs that have a reputation for immune enhancement, most commonly goldenseal. The usual dose of the liquid extract is twenty-five to sixty drops, two or three times daily.

Although some herbalists suggest taking it on a routine basis, the evidence more strongly supports the short-term use of echinacea at the start of an infection. Its effectiveness probably wanes after taking it for more than ten days in a row.

ECHINACEA AND AYURVEDA

Although not known to Ayurvedic physicians in India, echinacea can be understood as a potent detoxifying substance, similar in some ways to neem. It carries the bitter and pungent tastes and has a net cooling effect on the physiology. It is reducing to Pitta and Kapha, but can be aggravating to Vata if used for a prolonged period.

PRECAUTIONS

Most studies of neem emphasize its safety in both adults and children. A recent review stated the only adverse reactions were to the taste of the extract.[14] Echinacea has been shown to be virtually non-toxic to mice and rats.[15] However, a recent report from Australia identified a woman who may have had a severe allergic reaction to echinacea, and cautioned that people with a history of allergy may show a hypersensitivity to echinacea, even upon first exposure.[16]

Circulatory/Respiratory	Detoxifier	Digestive	Immune Enhancer	Men's Health
	X		X	
Metabolic	Nervine	Rejuvenative	Rheumatic	Women's Health

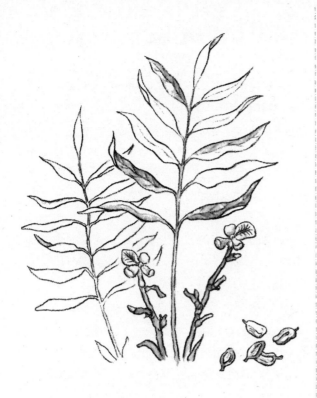

ELETTERIA CARDAMOMUM

FAMILIAR: **cardamom**
LATIN: *Eletteria cardamomum*
SANSKRIT: ela

For millennia the enticing, sweet, and pungent aroma of cardamom has been prized around the world. Described in the early Ayurvedic texts, valued by the ancient Greeks, and coveted by European powers during the Renaissance, cardamom has traditionally been associated with royalty and haute cuisine. The famous collection of stories known as *The Arabian Nights* is spiced with references to cardamom, a favorite Middle Eastern flavoring added to soften the bitterness of coffee. Both historically and today, this unique spice is highly sought after and relatively high-priced. Cardamom is the spice of celebrations and hospitality.

BOTANICAL AND PHYTOCHEMICAL INFORMATION

The cardamom plant, found in the tropical rain forests of India and growing wild on the coastal hills, is a perennial that grows up to ten feet high and bears a delicate yellowish white flower with violet stripes. The spice comes from the aromatic green seed pods, which can hold up to eighteen seeds. The pods are harvested before they ripen, and are sun-dried until they open and release the treasured seeds.

Up to 8 percent of a cardamom seed consists of an essential oil that contains a variety of volatile substances including limonene, cineol, terpineol, and terpinene.

THE SCIENCE OF CARDAMOM

Cardamom has received very little scientific attention for its medicinal qualities. Animal studies from Saudi Arabia have demonstrated that the steam-distilled oil has anti-inflammatory and pain-relieving properties.[1] It also reduces muscle spasms, acting on receptors for acetylcholine, the neurochemical that generates muscle contractions.

Studies from Asia have shown that cardamom oil enhances the penetration of other drugs through the skin. Mixing cardamom oil with the anti-inflammatory medicine indocin and with the steroid drug prednisolone increased the amount of the medicine that penetrated the skin.[2, 3] These effects may eventually be helpful in improving the delivery of dermatological medicines.

In a study from China, cardamom, along with other herbs, was reported to reduce the side effects of different chemotherapy drugs.[4] Cardamom's aromatic essential oil may help reduce nausea.

THE PRACTICAL USE OF CARDAMOM

Cardamom is best known as a culinary spice. It is considered a member of the sweet spices group and is commonly used to flavor candies and bakery goods. Cardamom is often added to curried spiced blends, rice pilafs, and pastries to provide its distinctive flavor and aroma. Although it is not as well known in American cooking, cardamom is an important spice in kitchens ranging from India to Africa, and from Arabia to South America. The essential oil extracted from the almost-ripe fruits is used in perfumes and to flavor coffees and liqueurs. Cardamom seeds can be chewed to sweeten the breath and are offered to guests at the end of a meal as a sign of hospitality.

Cardamom has been used medicinally for many health concerns. The generally soothing effects of the essential oil are applied to conditions affecting both the respiratory and digestive tracts. Cardamom tea or crushed seeds may be given to people with asthma to relieve respiratory spasms. Sinus congestion resulting from a cold may also respond to the aromatic properties of cardamom.

In the digestive system it is considered a carminative, useful in relieving gas and bloating. It enlivens the digestive fire and is usually well accepted by people with poor digestion who have difficulty tolerating the hotter spices such as ginger or cayenne. It has a very mild laxative effect and can be particularly helpful in relieving abdominal discomfort after overeating. When people transition from a meat-based diet to a primarily vegetarian one, they occasionally go through a phase of gaseousness and digestive irritability. Cardamom tea will often promptly alleviate the gastrointestinal stagnation. It can safely be given to children for mild stomach aches with a potency similar to chamomile.

Cardamom has a warming effect on the system, which can help with mild circulation problems characterized by cold hands and feet. It can also relieve chills when one is facing a cold or flu. Its pleasant taste makes it a good herb to combine with other, less appetizing ones in order to improve their palatability.

We recommend adding a pinch of cardamom powder to hot milk before bed as an aid to sound sleep. The combination of nutmeg, cardamom, and a teaspoon of brown sugar or honey enhances milk's relaxing effect. The cardamom also seems to improve the digestibility of milk in people who are sensitive to dairy. Cardamom is a good example of a spice that illustrates the close relationship between an herb's medicinal and culinary value.

HOW TO USE CARDAMOM

Cardamom is readily available as whole and ground seeds in most grocery, health food, and herb stores. It can be used singly or as part of a digestive formula consisting of equal parts ground cardamom seeds, cinnamon, and nutmeg. As a tea, place one-quarter to one-half teaspoon steeped in a cup of boiling water for ten minutes. This will create a weak infusion that can be sweetened or taken alone.

Cardamom seeds mix well with fennel seeds to soothe indigestion after overeating.

This mixture also makes a nice natural breath freshener. Cardamom mixed with a little grated gingerroot can help reduce nausea and may be helpful in pregnancy for morning sickness.

Adding one-quarter teaspoon of ground cardamom seed to your coffee will soften the bitterness and give you a taste of Arabia. Cardamom can also be combined with black tea, cloves, milk, and honey for a delicious and exotic fatigue reliever.

AYURVEDA AND CARDAMOM

From an Ayurvedic perspective, cardamom is a warming herb whose potential Pitta-aggravating qualities are balanced by its sweet taste. It can be used liberally by people with a Vata or Kapha constitution, and will not overstimulate Pitta except in high quantities.

PRECAUTIONS

Taken as a culinary spice, cardamom is very safe. Occasionally people with active peptic ulcers report mild digestive distress with high doses.

Circulatory/Respiratory	Detoxifier	Digestive	Immune Enhancer	Men's Health
X		X		
Metabolic	Nervine	Rejuvenative	Rheumatic	Women's Health
	X	X		

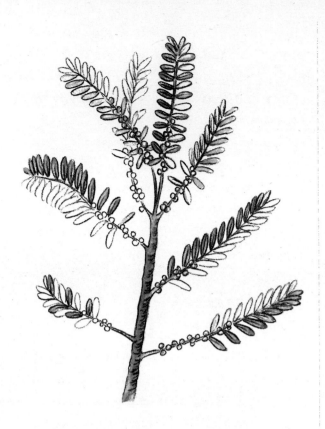

EMBLICA
OFFICINALIS

FAMILIAR: **amalaki, Indian gooseberry**
LATIN: *Emblica officinalis*
SANSKRIT: amalaki

Amalaki is considered the best herbal medicine for rejuvenation in Ayurveda. It can be used alone or in combination with many other herbs. The basis of the most famous Ayurvedic herbal jam, *Chavan Prash,* amalaki is considered capable of reversing the aging process. From a taste standpoint, it is among the most complicated edible substances, possessing five of the six basic flavors (lacking only the salty taste). Native to the forests of India, amalaki is valued throughout Nepal, Tibet, and the Middle East.

Amalaki is one of the richest natural sources of antioxidant vitamins, with its juice possessing almost twenty times as much vitamin C as orange juice. It has wide traditional uses, including the treatment of skin diseases, lung conditions, diabetes, and indigestion. It is one of the three ingredients of Triphala, the most important Ayurvedic bowel tonic.

BOTANICAL AND PHYTOCHEMICAL INFORMATION

Amalaki fruits are obtained from the *Emblica officinalis* tree, which grows in tropical and subtropical climates. The fruit is less than an inch in diameter and has a segmented appearance. Yellowish brown when fresh, the fruit turns nearly black as it dries. There is almost one gram of vitamin C in a half-cup of amalaki juice.[1] Small amounts of calcium, potassium, iron, and B vitamins are also present in the amalaki fruit. Many different tannins as well as pectin are constituents of amalaki.

THE SCIENCE OF AMALAKI

Amalaki's traditional role as a rejuvenating herbal medicine has been studied in two major health areas: cancer and heart disease. Studies in animals have suggested that amalaki may slow the development and growth of cancer cells. In a study from India, mice given a known cancer-causing chemical along with amalaki had significantly fewer harmful genetic changes than those given the carcinogen alone.[2] Amalaki has also been shown to reduce genetic mutations in bacteria exposed to substances that have been identified to cause cancer.[3]

An herbal jam made with amalaki, called MAK-4, has been studied in several animal models. In one study it was found to inhibit cancerous changes induced by a toxic chemical.[4] In another it was found to reduce both the number and size of metastatic cancerous lesions.[5] The relevance of these reports to human cancers remains to be clarified, but the preliminary results are encouraging.

The other major area of scientific interest in amalaki is its role in the lowering of serum cholesterol levels. Several studies in rabbits have shown that amalaki is effective in reducing blood cholesterol values and the deposition of fat into blood vessels.[6, 7] In a study in rabbits, amalaki reduced serum cholesterol levels by over 80 percent.[8]

This cholesterol-lowering effect is applicable to human beings as well. Men whose diet was supplemented with amalaki for one month demonstrated lowering of their serum cholesterol levels, whether or not their cholesterol was elevated before they began taking the amalaki.[9] Other studies have suggested that amalaki-based supplements can reduce the harmful oxidation of cholesterol in men.[10] It may also decrease the stickiness of platelets, lowering the risk of unwanted blood clotting.[11]

Other potential therapeutic effects of amalaki have received preliminary scientific attention. It has been used traditionally in the treatment of heartburn, and one report has provided some support for this use.[12] It also has a reputation for the treatment of liver and pancreatic conditions, and in one animal study it was able to reduce the extent of tissue damage caused by experimental pancreatitis.[13] Although amalaki has classically been recommended in the treatment of diabetes mellitus, there has been no scientific research to evaluate this use. Studies have shown that amalaki does have antibiotic activity against a wide range of bacteria, possibly explaining its traditional role in the treatment of lung infections.[14]

THE PRACTICAL USE OF AMALAKI

Amalaki forms the basis of the premier Ayurvedic rejuvenative jam traditionally known as *Chavan Prash,* named after the doctor who developed the formula thousands of years ago. We recommend this mixture of amalaki fruit with many other tonic herbs for people recovering from illness as well as for those seeking rejuvenation. A teaspoon twice daily is the usual dosage, either taken straight or mixed in juice or warm milk.

Amalaki is also readily available in Triphala, the gentle Ayurvedic bowel tonic that can be helpful in people with chronic constipation as well as those with irritable bowel syndrome. Mixed with shatavari, fennel, and turmeric, it can be effective in reducing hyperacidity.

As a cholesterol agent, amalaki combines well with guggulu. This same combination may be helpful in diabetes, rheumatic conditions, and liver ailments.

HOW TO USE AMALAKI

As a component of triphala, amalaki represents one-third of a typical half-gram tablet. The usual dose to improve colon function is one to two grams daily in divided doses. As a treatment for elevated cholesterol, begin with one gram twice daily. In the form of amalaki herbal jam, a teaspoon morning and evening will provide you with a good dose of this potent herbal antioxidant.

AYURVEDA AND AMALAKI

Although the sweet taste predominates in amalaki, its complex nature makes it appropriate for all three doshas. Because it is a rich rasayana, whenever possible it is advisable to first undergo a period of detoxification before taking amalaki. It is traditionally considered to be rejuvenating for Pitta imbalances, and strengthening to the liver, stomach, heart, and blood.

PRECAUTIONS

Owing to its laxative qualities, amalaki should be used carefully in people with a tendency toward loose bowels. Many herbal jam formulations of amalaki have high concentrations of sugar and clarified butter (ghee). Chavan Prash should therefore be used carefully by people with diabetes and high cholesterol; without the sugar and ghee, amalaki is considered helpful for these conditions.

Circulatory/Respiratory	Detoxifier	Digestive	Immune Enhancer	Men's Health
X		X	X	X
Metabolic	Nervine	Rejuvenative	Rheumatic	Women's Health
		X	X	

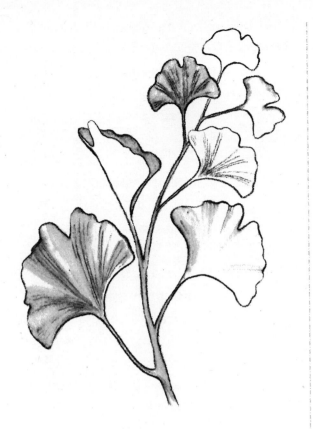

GINKGO
BILOBA

FAMILIAR: **ginkgo**
LATIN: *ginkgo biloba*

Ginkgo may be the most ancient tree on earth, dating back 200 million years. Once found in North America and Europe, it survived only in China after the prehistoric ice ages. Prized for its medicinal properties for almost five thousand years, ginkgo is now one of the most popular herbs in Europe and the United States. The name *ginkgo* is

derived from the Japanese words *gin,* meaning "silver" and *kyo* meaning "apricot," referring to the inedible fruits that appear in the summer.

Serious interest in ginkgo has been expanding in the West over the past quarter-century as scientific research has documented the therapeutic benefits of this ancient herb on circulation, memory, hearing, and balance. A dry extract of ginkgo called EGb (extract of *Ginkgo biloba*) is now the standardized herbal product that is receiving attention around the world.

BOTANICAL
AND PHYTOCHEMICAL
INFORMATION

Ginkgo is a deciduous tree that can grow to heights of over one hundred feet and may live as long as one thousand years. Originally cultivated in China, ginkgo trees are now grown on farms in Japan, France, and, most recently, the southeastern United States. It is a remarkably hardy plant, tolerant of pollution and pests, and able to thrive in modern urban environments.

The characteristic fanlike leaves of ginkgo have two lobes, accounting for its species name, *biloba*. The leaves are harvested in the fall and put through an extraction process using an acetone-and-water mixture. The solvent is removed and the extract is standardized to yield 24 percent flavone glycosides and 5 to 7 percent terpene lactones. These compounds have a variety of pharmacological effects, including antioxidant, circulation-enhancing, and nerve-cells-protective action. Ginkgo extract also inhibits a natural substance called platelet activation factor (PAF) that is an important component of the clotting system. The various properties of ginkgo may combine to explain its clinical value in improving memory and circulation.

THE SCIENCE OF GINKGO

Hundreds of scientific studies have been published on the laboratory and clinical effects of ginkgo. It is a complex medicinal substance whose full range of properties have yet to be characterized. It has diverse actions, including the ability to protect cell membranes, neutralize free radicals, protect tissues from oxygen deprivation, and improve circulation. Because it appears to have very few side effects, medical researchers have been performing clinical studies to test the applicability of the laboratory and animal findings to people.

Initial studies on ginkgo in human beings focused on its ability to enhance blood supply to the brain as well as to increase the brain's ability to utilize oxygen and energy sources.[1, 2] Ginkgo extract has also been shown to protect the integrity of nerve cells deprived of oxygen.[3] These initial findings led to a number of clinical studies in people with impaired neurological functioning believed to result from lack of circulation to the brain. At the time of many of these studies, memory impairment was often blamed on lack of blood supply, and improving circulation to the brain was believed to help people think more clearly. Several reports of people given ginkgo demonstrated that they performed better on tests of mental functioning.[4, 5]

We have since learned that most elderly people with serious memory problems have a degenerative condition such as Alzheimer's disease or multiple small strokes rather than a generalized lack of blood supply to the brain. Recent studies have evaluated the role of ginkgo in patients with these conditions and found that it can provide definite value. A small German study found that people with Alzheimer's disease taking 240 milligrams of ginkgo extract per day showed improvement in their mental functioning compared with a deterioration in those taking a placebo.[6] A larger study of people with dementia resulting either from Alzheimer's disease or multiple small strokes also found that ginkgo improved their memory and quality of life.[7] A recent North American study also found that people with dementia taking ginkgo did not deteriorate as quickly as those on a placebo and in a number of cases actually improved.[8] Although the benefits have generally been mild to moderate, these are nonetheless remarkable findings, for there has been very little else to offer patients with this devastating condition. The currently available pharmacological agents are not very effective, have substantial side effects, and are very expensive.

Does ginkgo provide any memory benefit to people without brain diseases? We do not yet know the answer to this question. Mice given ginkgo learn more quickly, with less anxiety, but we do not know if this has relevance in people.[9] Of interest is the finding that mice receiving ginkgo show subtle changes in nerve cells that reside in the memory center of their brain, providing a possible anatomical explanation for the observed enhancement of memory.[10] A study of basically healthy people with fatigue found that those taking ginkgo in combination with ginseng scored slightly higher on tests of cognitive function than those taking a placebo.[11] Although we do not recommend that everyone take ginkgo as a brain food, it does appear to provide a safe approach for those having difficulty maintaining their mental focus.

In addition to the memory-enhancing effects of ginkgo, this ancient botanical medicine has shown many other potentially beneficial health effects. A common condition that develops as people age is impaired circulation to the legs, which results in pain when walking. Some studies, but not all, have shown that ginkgo may benefit this condition, known as intermittent claudication. Reports from Germany found that patients taking ginkgo are able to walk farther with less pain than those taking a placebo.[12, 13] Another study from Denmark did not find improvement in the ambulatory capacity of people taking ginkgo, but did find that these patients had improved concentration and memory.[14]

Ginkgo has been tested in the treatment of hearing and balance problems and found to have potential benefit. Cats with damage to their balance systems showed faster recoveries if ginkgo was added to their diet, while guinea pigs exposed to loud noises and given ginkgo had less damage to their hearing nerves than those left untreated.[15, 16] A study in people with episodes of dizziness and ringing in their ears demonstrated some improvement in both symptoms after taking ginkgo for several months.[17]

A potentially important application of ginkgo is in the prevention of mountain sickness. In a report from France, mountain climbers on a Himalayan expedition who took ginkgo weathered the high altitude much better than their colleagues given a placebo.[18] None of the subjects hiking to over fifteen thousand feet taking ginkgo developed acute brain mountain sickness, compared to over 40 percent in the control group. Breathing problems were six times as likely in climbers who took a placebo as in those on ginkgo. The mountain climbers on ginkgo also had fewer problems with the blood vessel changes that lead to frostbite.

Ginkgo has also been used in the treatment of asthma, with studies showing it can reduce the severity of wheezing caused by exercise, dust, and pollen.[19] One of ginkgo's pharmacological effects is to inhibit a natural inflammatory chemical called platelet activating factor (PAF), which has been implicated in asthma and allergies.

Another potential use for ginkgo is in the treatment of sexual dysfunction associated with antidepressant medications. Although the new antidepressant medicines are often very effective in improving mood, they may cause sexual dysfunction in both men and women. A recent report from San Francisco found that ginkgo was effective in improving all four phases of the sexual response (desire, excitement, orgasm, and resolution) in 91 percent of women and 76 percent of men.[20] Considering the recent frenzy created by Viagra, further testing of ginkgo is warranted in people with sexual potency problems from all causes to see if this safe herbal medicine may be of value.

Ginkgo has been studied in the treatment of ulcerative colitis, anxiety, and premenstrual syndrome.[21–23] It may help enhance immune function, reduce oxida-tive stress during coronary artery surgery, and improve recovery after spinal cord injury.[24–26] It is obvious that this ancient tree has evolved a vast pharmacy of natural healing substances that we have just begun to appreciate in modern times.

THE PRACTICAL USE OF GINKGO

Most people who use ginkgo have concerns about their memory. This may show up as difficulty with concentration, trouble recalling names, or simple forgetfulness. Most of the time these minor concerns do not represent a serious neurological condition, and it is reasonable to try ginkgo for a few months before undergoing a formal memory evaluation. If someone has been diagnosed with Alzheimer's disease, a trial of ginkgo is warranted under the supervision of a physician who is familiar with this illness.

The use of ginkgo in intermittent claudication should be discussed with your doctor to be certain that other treatments are not more appropriate. For symptoms of dizziness or ringing in the ears, be certain to have a medical evaluation to rule out treatable specific causes before starting ginkgo. The risks of taking ginkgo for sexual dysfunction are very low, but we recommend you discuss its use with your health-care provider if you are taking any prescribed medications.

How to Use Ginkgo

Ginkgo products in the United States have followed the lead of European manufacturers with almost all tablets and capsules standardized to 24 percent flavone glycosides and 6 percent terpene lactones. The ginkgo extract usually represents a 50:1 concentration that provides 40 or 60 milligrams per tablet. Most studies have used between 120 and 320 milligrams on a daily basis in divided doses.

When you first begin ginkgo, start with 120 milligrams per day, in two or three divided doses. Wait at least a month to assess the effects before gradually increasing the dose by 40 milligrams per day.

Ayurveda and Ginkgo

Despite its ancient Asian heritage, ginkgo was not described in the ancient Ayurvedic texts. Its properties are similar to the Ayurvedic herb gotu kola. The predominant taste of ginkgo extract is bitter, with a minor sour component. It can be balancing to all three doshas and has a net cooling effect on the physiology.

Precautions

Although rare, headaches and mild digestive upset can occur in people taking ginkgo. The headache is usually mild and can be minimized by starting with a low dose. There have been two case reports of people developing bleeding complications while on ginkgo. One involved bleeding into the eye in a seventy-year-old man who had been taking aspirin.[27] The other was a case of a young woman on ginkgo for two years who developed blood clots on her brain.[28] No obvious explanation for the bleeding could be uncovered. Although these possible complications are exceedingly rare, it is recommended not to take ginkgo if you have any type of bleeding condition or are taking any blood-thinning medication, including aspirin.

Circulatory/Respiratory	Detoxifier	Digestive	Immune Enhancer	Men's Health
X				
Metabolic	Nervine	Rejuvenative	Rheumatic	Women's Health
	X			X

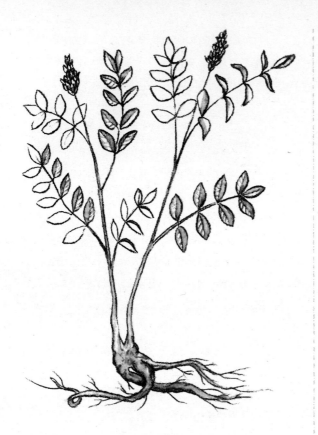

GLYCYRRHIZA GLABRA

FAMILIAR: **licorice**
LATIN: *Glycyrrhiza glabra*
SANSKRIT: yasthimadhu

The chewy black candy that many of us loved as children is derived from the roots of a plant long treasured by healing cultures across Asia, Europe, and the Mediterranean. In addition to providing a sweet flavoring that is fifty times more intense than sugar, licorice contains a number of therapeutic medici-

nal substances. It has many potential uses in conditions of the digestive and respiratory systems. Its intensely sweet taste makes licorice an ideal additive to disguise other, less palatable medicines and herbs. Its name in Sanskrit, *yasthimadhu,* means "stick of sweetness."

Honored for thousands of years as a treatment for inflammatory conditions, modern studies have documented that licorice has steroidlike actions. Used cautiously and with respect, licorice is a valuable healing plant, but at excessive levels it can cause potentially dangerous side effects.

BOTANICAL AND PHYTOCHEMICAL INFORMATION

The shrub from which licorice is derived is a member of the legume family. This perennial plant produces small, pealike blue flowers and may reach six feet in height. The roots are harvested and processed to yield a sugary paste that is used as a flavoring for candy and medicine.

Licorice contains a number of chemical compounds including phytoestrogens, sugars, and flavonoids. The most investigated component of licorice is glycyrrhizic acid. This substance seems to be responsible for many of licorice's anti-inflammatory properties through mechanisms that have only recently been unraveled. It appears that in the digestive tract, glycyrrhizic acid is converted into glycyrrhetic acid. This chemical inhibits the enzyme that metabolizes the natural steroid cortisol, resulting in higher circulating levels of this steroid, with its known anti-inflammatory effects.

The downside of licorice's steroidlike actions is the potential for elevated blood pressure, because it can cause the body to retain too much sodium. For this reason, the medicinal use of licorice must be moderate and carefully monitored. Licorice contains many other natural chemicals, including components with estrogenlike effects, immune stimulating activity, and antiviral properties.

THE SCIENCE OF LICORICE

Hundreds of scientific studies have been published on licorice, documenting its potent physiological properties. It is a strong anti-inflammatory substance that reduces pain and fever. Although its actions are related to cortisol and hydrocortisone, it does not cause ulcers in the digestive tract or suppress the production of blood cells as standard steroids do.[1] Components of licorice function as powerful antioxidants that may be helpful in reducing both heart disease and cancer.[2, 3]

Laboratory studies paint a complex picture of the pharmacological properties of licorice. Licorice appears to reduce elevated cholesterol levels and to prolong the clotting time of blood.[4, 5] These combined effects could be beneficial in patients at risk for coronary artery disease. One possible explanation of how licorice works is that it stimulates enzymes in the liver that neutralize toxic substances from the environment.[6]

A potentially important use for licorice is in the treatment of viral infections. Studies have reported that licorice has the ability to inactivate a wide range of different viruses.[7] Reports from Japan have suggested that licorice can have a beneficial impact on people with chronic hepatitis B infection.[8] Glycyrrhizin can stimulate the production of the potent immune-enhancing substance interferon and is capable of enhancing the activity of key immune cells.[9, 10]

The medicinal applications of licorice in people are still being explored. One of its traditional uses has been in the treatment of peptic ulcers, and animal studies have shown that licorice stimulates the production of protective mucus in the stomach lining.[11] Studies from over forty years ago demonstrated that licorice extracts could promote the healing of ulcers.[12] Concerns about side effects and the development of acid secretion blocking agents has essentially eliminated the role of licorice in the mainstream therapy of ulcers in the United

States, although it remains in comparatively wide use for this purpose in Europe.

Taking advantage of its blood-pressure-raising potential, researchers have employed licorice in the treatment of low blood pressure caused by diabetes mellitus.[13] It has also been of benefit in the treatment of low blood pressure that is sometimes associated with chronic fatigue syndrome.[14]

Although there is a legitimate concern about the side effects of licorice, most complications occur in people taking excessive doses. Elevated blood pressure has been reported in men consuming 50 grams of licorice candy daily, which corresponds to a dosage of between 100 to 200 milligrams of glycyrrhizic acid.[15] Other reports have suggested that people do not show any ill effects from licorice until their daily intake of glycyrrhizic acid approaches 400 milligrams for two weeks.[16] To stay within a safe range, do not consume more than 100 milligrams of glycyrrhizic acid per day. This usually means taking no more than 2.5 grams of dried licorice root on a daily basis and not using it continuously for more than four to six weeks at a time.

THE PRACTICAL USE OF LICORICE

Licorice has traditionally been used in the treatment of coughs and colds to help mobilize secretions. A tea composed of equal parts licorice and fresh ginger provides the right balance of pungency and smoothness to loosen and discharge mucus. Mixed with amalaki and shatavari, it is useful in the treatment of heartburn and hyperacidity. A strong infusion made with licorice root and slippery elm is a useful soothing gargle or mouthwash for sore throats and canker sores.

We occasionally prescribe licorice to reduce the accumulated heat in women experiencing hot flashes during menopause. Its mild laxative action can contribute to the efficacy of Triphala. For people trying to lose weight or stop smoking, we suggest that they suck on natural licorice-root sticks, which can satisfy oral cravings.

For people suffering with chronic fatigue, a daily cup of licorice tea may prove helpful in generating vitality when taken upon awakening in the morning. In other conditions where a person may be trying to decrease his or her steroid requirement in conditions such as chronic bronchitis or asthma, a cup of licorice-and-ginger tea two to three times daily may tip the balance in favor of less medication. Be certain to work closely with your health-care adviser if you are using licorice more than occasionally.

HOW TO USE LICORICE

Bulk chopped licorice root is available at most health-food stores. A tablespoon of the chopped roots or a teaspoon of the shredded roots in a cup of hot water makes a moderately strong tea. The addition of one-quarter teaspoon of powdered licorice root to bitter herbs makes them much more palatable.

Powdered licorice in the form of capsules can be taken in doses up to 2.5 grams per day. Most of the major herbal companies have standardized the glycyrrhizic acid content of their licorice capsules. Check the amount per capsule, and limit your total daily intake to 100 milligrams. The German Commission E recommends limiting a course of licorice to no longer than six weeks at a time.

AYURVEDA AND LICORICE

Licorice is predominantly sweet and bitter, with a cooling effect. Although, with its sweet taste and cooling potency, one might not anticipate its value in Kapha conditions such as upper respiratory congestion, its special properties of loosening and mobilizing mucus outweigh its potential Kapha-augmenting effects. Its heavy, sweet smoothness is balancing to Vata, while its cooling influence makes licorice particularly useful for balancing aggravated Pitta.

PRECAUTIONS

Do not take licorice if you have elevated blood pressure or are taking diuretic medications. Be certain that you do not exceed the safe recommended dose. Most licorice root contains between 4 and 8 percent glycyrrhizic acid, so a 500-milligram tablet of the dried powdered root will have 20 to 40 milligrams. Do not take unnecessary risks with this herb.

Circulatory/Respiratory	Detoxifier	Digestive	Immune Enhancer	Men's Health
X		X	X	
Metabolic	*Nervine*	*Rejuvenative*	*Rheumatic*	*Women's Health*
			X	

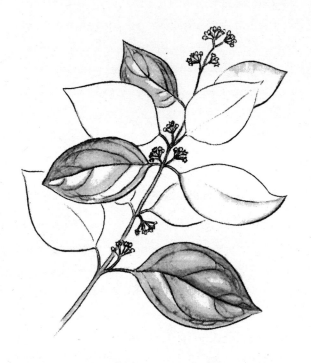

GYMNEMA
SYLVESTRE

FAMILIAR: **gurmar**
LATIN: *Gymnema sylvestre*
SANSKRIT/HINDI: mehasringi,
gurmar

Gurmar is a fascinating example of an herb that complies with the "doctrine of signatures." This ancient precept postulates that nature intentionally provides clues to the medicinal value of an herb. When the leaves of gur-mar are chewed, the tongue becomes insensitive to the taste of sweetness for about an hour. This effect is the origin of the Hindi word for this herb, *gurmar,* meaning "destroyer of sweet." Ayurvedic doctors reasoned that if this plant neutralized the effects of sugar on the tongue, it might have a similar action in the body. Consequently it was given to people with diabetes mellitus and found effective in reducing the symptoms of this common metabolic condition. Many modern studies have confirmed a therapeutic influence of gurmar on sugar metabolism.

BOTANICAL AND PHYTOCHEMICAL INFORMATION

Gymnema sylvestre is a climbing plant commonly found in the southern and central parts of India. It has one-inch-long elliptical leaves and small yellow flowers. The leaves are the source of many unique phytochemicals, six of which have been characterized as gymnemic acids. Many triterpene glycosides and triterpenoid saponins have been identified in gurmar, which may contribute to its glucose-regulating properties. A sweetness-suppressing polypeptide called gurmarin, consisting of thirty-five amino acids, appears to fold itself into a three-dimensional structure that binds with the sweet taste receptor, blocking the effects of sugar on the tongue.[1] The chemicals responsible for gurmar's effects on sugar metabolism in the body remain to be characterized.

THE SCIENCE OF GURMAR

Diabetes mellitus is a common and often disabling illness affecting almost 16 million Americans. It is a condition in which sugar is not normally managed, resulting in higher blood glucose levels. Diabetes can be caused by inadequate production of insulin by cells in the pancreas (Type I) or by a decreased sensitivity of cells to insulin (Type II). Chronically elevated blood sugars can lead to kidney, nerve, eye, and blood vessel damage; therefore, good control of diabetes is essential to reducing the risk of disabling complications. The appropriate use of supplemental insulin and oral agents has led to marked improvements in the lives of people with diabetes. Gurmar may be another useful agent in therapy of this prevalent illness.

Studies in animals have shown that gurmar has many different effects on the metabolism of sugar. One of the most consistent findings is the reduction of glucose absorption from the digestive tract in animals given gurmar. Chemicals in gurmar inhibit the uptake of sugar from the small intestines resulting in a lowering of blood sugar levels.[2, 3] In addition to blocking sugar absorption, gurmar extracts have also been shown to inhibit the absorption of oleic acid, a building block of fat in the body.[4]

Gurmar has other interesting effects on glucose metabolism. Components of gurmar slow the uptake of glucose into muscles and inhibit the storage of glycogen in the liver.[5, 6] Absorption of cholesterol is also reduced.[7] The net effect of these various actions is better sugar tolerance. Diabetic rats fed daily doses of gurmar extracts showed lower blood sugar levels, higher insulin levels, and a doubling in the number of cells in the pancreas responsible for producing insulin.[8] If these findings are applicable to people, gurmar could be an important advance in the treatment of diabetes mellitus.

Although formal studies in human beings are limited, initial reports are encouraging. Patients with insulin-dependent diabetes given a daily dose of a gurmar extract had a reduction in their insulin requirements and a lowering of their fasting glucose levels.[9] Diabetic patients who did not require insulin also benefited from gurmar, showing a reduction in their blood sugar levels and a reduced need for their oral diabetic medicines.[10] Five of the twenty-two patients in the study were able to completely discontinue their medications, maintaining control solely with gurmar. These reports are intriguing and warrant further studies to define the appropriate role for gurmar in the treatment of diabetes.

Another application for this herb is in the treatment of obesity. Neuro-physiological studies have found that when gurmar is present on the tongue, taste nerves fail to send the information about sweetness to the brain.[11] Along with its effect on decreasing the absorption of sugar from the digestive tract, gurmar could be a helpful nutritional aid to reduce the cravings and caloric load of people with obesity. The possible value of gurmar in reducing caloric intake was tested by a small study that found that people given *Gymnema sylvestre* prior to a snack meal ate less total calories than those that did not take the herb.[12] A study from the 1960s suggested that gurmar actually led to an increase in the weight of rats, but this has not been reported in human beings.[13] Given the rising incidence of obesity in this culture and the relative lack of success of most weight-loss programs, gurmar may represent a valuable adjunct to a balanced nutritional and exercise program for people trying to shed excessive pounds.

THE PRACTICAL USE OF GURMAR

Gurmar is currently available from a few major herbal suppliers. If you are wishing to use it as an aid in a weight-loss program, try placing a pinch on your tongue, fifteen minutes before your meal or whenever you find yourself about to indulge in a sweet craving that you know is not in your best interest. In the Perfect Weight programs at the Chopra Center, we recommend that our participants take a taste of gurmar before their main meals and swallow a capsule with each meal.

If you have diabetes mellitus and are using gurmar as a blood-sugar-lowering agent, be certain to discuss its use with your health-care provider before adding it to your diet. Because gurmar has been shown to have measurable blood-glucose-lowering effects, you must closely monitor your blood sugar levels to quantify its effects and adjust your other medications accordingly.

Be sure to pay attention to the other essential components of a healthy mind-body program, including a balanced diet, regular exercise, and listening carefully to your internal signals of hunger and satiety. Do not rely on gurmar as the sole approach to balancing your metabolism. View it as a short-term ally as you establish long-term healthy practices.

HOW TO USE GURMAR

Gurmar is available in 450-milligram capsules, standardized to 150 milligrams of gymnemic acids. For weight control, try breaking open a tablet and placing a small amount on your tongue. Notice how your craving for sweetness is altered as a result of the change in your taste sensations. Ingest the rest of the capsule with your meal. Do not take more than two doses per day while monitoring your food intake.

If you have diabetes, first consult with your health-care adviser and make the commitment to closely monitor your blood sugar levels. Begin with one dose in the morning and see how you feel and what your glucose levels do. Wait at least two weeks before increasing your dose to twice daily, before breakfast and in the late afternoon. Watch closely for any signs that your blood sugar is getting too low.

AYURVEDA AND GURMAR

According to Ayurveda, gurmar carries astringent and pungent flavors with a net heating effect on the physiology. It is pacifying to Kapha and essentially neutral to Pitta and Vata.

In addition to its long-standing role in the treatment of diabetes, gurmar has also been used in Ayurveda in the treatment of upper respiratory infections and fevers. Applied topically to skin infections, a paste of gurmar is used to draw out infection.

PRECAUTIONS

Although there have not been reports of serious hypoglycemic reactions, you should be alert to the possibility, especially if you are taking blood-sugar-lowering medications. A problem with the regular application of gurmar to the tongue is that sweetly flavored foods become less palatable. Therefore, use gurmar to add motivation to your weight-loss program, but put your attention on developing good nutritional habits so that you can maintain your appropriate weight through healthy diet and activity.

Circulatory/Respiratory	Detoxifier	Digestive	Immune Enhancer	Men's Health
Metabolic	Nervine	Rejuvenative	Rheumatic	Women's Health
X				

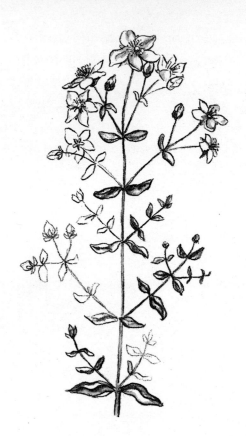

HYPERICUM
PERFORATUM

FAMILIAR: **St. John's wort, hypericum**
LATIN: *Hypericum perforatum*

O f all the herbs in the modern botanical medicine chest, few can rival hypericum's meteoric rise to fame. It has received enthusiastic reception from the lay public and grudging acceptance from the scientific medical community. As a generally safe and effective natural remedy for the treatment of mild to moderate depression, St. John's wort offers an alternative to the standard antidepressant medications. It is readily available and inexpensive, and carries minimal risk.

The origin of the name St. John's wort (*wort* is from Middle English for "plant") is clouded in the mists of myth and history. Some believe the name was applied because hypericum blooms in late June, around the time that John the Baptist's birthday is celebrated. Others say its name was a reference to the red juice from its petals, which presumably symbolized the blood of St. John. However it acquired its name, St. John's wort has been an honored medicinal plant since the time of the ancient Greeks. Popular during the Middle Ages, it has a traditional use in the treatment of a wide range of psychic and physical ailments, from melancholy to varicose veins.

BOTANICAL AND PHYTOCHEMICAL INFORMATION

Hypericum grows wild throughout Europe and the United States. It is a perennial, sun-loving plant that grows up to three feet in height. During the summer months it produces numerous yellow flowers with five petals that are marked with small black dots and lines. The flowering tops and leaves of St. John's wort are the source of the medicinal constituents that are the object of intense scientific interest.

Chemical analysis of hypericum reveals many different components including naphthodianthrones, phloroglucinols, flavonoids, phenylpropanes, proanthocyanidins, and amino acids. The most important medicinally active ingredients, which are extracted in methanol, are found in the naphthodianthrone and phloroglucinol portions. The natural chemicals that account for hypericum's antidepressant activity are not yet fully sorted out. Hypericin, a naphthodianthrone, has been the leading candidate for several years, and almost all commercially available St. John's wort is standardized to yield a .3 percent extract. However, several recent studies have suggested that a phloroglucinol chemical called hyperforin is the most likely constituent responsible for the antidepressant actions of St. John's wort.[1, 2] This unique chemical influences several important brain neurochemicals that have been associated with mood and emotions.

THE SCIENCE OF ST. JOHN'S WORT

Almost half a century ago it was discovered that people given certain drugs experienced an improvement in their moods. Subsequent research to identify the biochemical correlates of depression has led to important discoveries about how the brain functions in health and illness. We now know that antidepressant medications work by restoring the balance of neurotransmitter molecules in the brain.

Chemicals found in St. John's wort have a significant influence on the levels of many important brain chemicals. Recent studies on hyperforin have shown that it increases the levels of serotonin, norepinephrine, and dopamine by blocking their reuptake by nerve cells.[3] It also influences other brain chemicals, including GABA and glutamate.[4]

Other components of St. John's wort may also play a role in its antidepressant effects. Until very recently, hypericin was felt to be the active ingredient and was thought to possibly act by inhibiting one of the enzymes that breaks down norepinephrine, called monoamine oxidase (MAO).[5] More recent studies, however, have suggested that at usual therapeutic doses, there are insufficient levels of hypericin levels to interfere with MAO.[6, 7] Other components of St. John's wort may bind to the same anti-anxiety receptors in the brain as the common tranquilizing drugs such as Valium do.[8]

Regardless of exactly how St. John's wort exerts its effects, there is convincing evidence in support of its antidepressant efficacy. More than twenty-five studies have evaluated the effects of hypericum on depression as compared with a placebo or a standard antidepressant medication, with most showing the benefit of St. John's wort. A meta-analysis that evaluated twenty-three randomized clinical trials concluded that St. John's wort was more effective than a placebo for mild to moderate depression, with only minor side effects.[9] Compared with the older tricyclic antidepressant medications, including imipramine and amitriptyline, hypericum was equally effective with fewer adverse reactions.[10, 11] In addition to a reduction in their depressive symptoms, people taking St. John's wort usually show less anxiety and improved sleep. Overall, between 60 and 80 percent of people respond to St. John's wort with some improvement in their mood.[12, 13] Hypericum has not yet been studied in comparison to the newer selective serotonin reuptake inhibitor (SSRI) antidepressant medications such as fluoxetine (Prozac) or sertraline (Zoloft).

A recent report found hypericum to be useful in the condition known as seasonal affective disorder or SAD. People with SAD become depressed during the winter months when there are fewer daylight hours, and one of the popular treatments for SAD is exposure to bright lights for a couple of hours each morning. A study of 168 people from England found that people taking St. John's wort had less anxiety, improved libido, and better sleep, whether or not they also received phototherapy.[14]

Although scientific research has been limited, hypericum has other potentially therapeutic properties. It has been shown to have antiviral and antibacterial activity in laboratory studies.[15–17] Components of hypericum may function as antioxidants and suppress inflammation.[18, 19] Anticancer effects have also been suggested for St. John's wort.[20, 21] Although we do not know if any of these potential effects will prove to be of benefit in people, it is reassuring to know that there may be positive side effects to taking hypericum.

THE PRACTICAL USE OF ST. JOHN'S WORT

It is very important to remember that depression is potentially serious, even life-threatening. If you are experiencing persistent sad thoughts or have even entertained the idea of committing suicide, seek professional help immediately. Hypericum seems to provide the greatest benefit for people with mild to moderate depression, but it will not magically elevate your mood. A beneficial effect may take up to six weeks to be apparent, so patience is required. Although some reports have suggested that higher doses of hypericum may benefit people who do not respond to lower ones, we do not recommend going beyond the standard recommendations unless you are under the care of a knowledgeable doctor.[22] The safety of St. John's wort taken along with standard antidepressant medications has not yet been adequately studied, so do not mix hypericum with your existing drug, except under the supervision of your physician. Also, do not stop your anti-depressant or anti-anxiety medicines without first discussing the matter with your health-care provider.

HOW TO USE HYPERICUM

Most hypericum products contain 300 milligrams of hypericum extract, standardized to deliver .3 percent hypericin, so that each dose delivers .9 milligrams. Unfortunately, studies have shown that many available compounds deliver substantially less than claimed on the label. In a recent *Los Angeles Times* investigation, most capsules or tablets delivered 20 to 90 percent of the stated amount, although products by two companies, Nature's Herbs and Natures Resource, actually delivered more than the label stated.[23] For a complete review of this issue, check out the hypericum Web site at **www.hypericum.com.**

The usual dose of St. John's wort is 300 milligrams three times daily, equivalent to a daily hypericin intake of 2.7 milligrams. As noted earlier, some reports have suggested that a higher daily intake, of 600 milligrams of hypericum extract three times daily, may provide additional benefit. With recent information that hyperforin rather than hypericin is the most important antidepressant component of St. John's wort, it makes more sense for

herbal manufacturers to standardize the newly defined chemical constituent.

Although there are liquid extracts of hypericum, we prefer the standardized solid extracts. It may be discovered that more than one component is important in St. John's wort, and you are less likely to miss one if you take a product that is closer to the whole herb.

It may take as long as six weeks to experience a therapeutic benefit. We often see people who tried hypericum for a short time at less than the recommended dose without noticing any benefit, but when they took it regularly at the prescribed level, a therapeutic effect was seen. If you do not see improvement after four to six weeks, discuss your condition with your health-care provider for other medical options, including prescribed medication.

PRECAUTIONS

When St. John's wort was believed to act by inhibiting the enzyme monoamine oxidase (MAO), warnings were sounded about potential side effects in people ingesting certain substances while taking the herb. Adverse reactions can occur with MAO-inhibitor antidepressant medications when people eat aged cheeses, dried sausages, alcohol, or stimulant drugs, because they contain substances that potentiate the effect of the medicines. Although there has been only one reported case of a possible reaction in a woman taking hypericum along with a stimulant drug for a bladder problem, it is prudent not to combine St. John's wort with MAO-inhibiting antidepressants or stimulant drugs.

Another commonly discussed potential complication of St. John's wort is photosensitivity. Sunlight can change hypericum molecules in the skin, provoking an allergic reaction. Although photosensitivity is often talked about, it has only been reported once in a woman who had been taking St. John's wort for three years.[24] The skin reaction rapidly subsided when hypericum was discontinued.

Other adverse reactions are generally mild and include digestive disturbances, fatigue, headache, and restlessness. In most studies, minor side effects are seen as often in people taking a placebo as those on St. John's wort. It is a relatively rare person who needs to discontinue the herb because of side effects.

Do not take St. John's wort if you are pregnant, because safety studies have not been done to determine whether it poses any risks to the unborn child. Do not take St. John's wort along with any prescription medication without first discussing it with your health-care provider.

Circulatory/Respiratory	Detoxifier	Digestive	Immune Enhancer	Men's Health
Metabolic	Nervine	Rejuvenative	Rheumatic	Women's Health
	X			

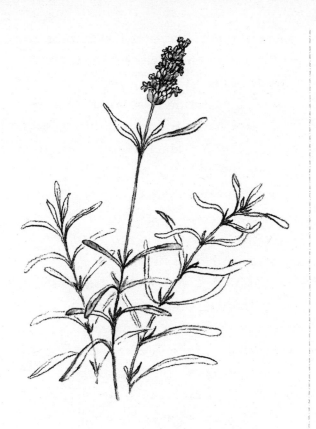

LAVANDULA
ANGUSTIFOLIA

FAMILIAR: **lavender**
LATIN: *Lavandula angustifolia*

The sweet and pungent beckoning aroma of lavender reminds us of its romantic history. The early Romans used lavender to scent their baths, providing us with the explanation for this fragrant herb's name, which is derived from the Latin *lavare,* meaning "to wash." Native to the Mediterranean, lavender was prized by the ancient Egyptians and

Turks. When brought to Europe, it found its way into churches and monasteries, where its pure aroma was believed to ward off evil spirits and disease-causing agents. For thousands of years lavender has been a popular herb used in perfumes, soaps, and sachets.

Lavender's color, pleasant aroma, and delicate flowers contributed to its long-standing reputation as a promoter of romance and dreamy tranquillity. Modern studies have demonstrated that many of lavender's traditional uses are based upon scientifically verifiable effects. Components of lavender carry antiseptic properties, while its leaves, flowers, and essential oil have a documented calming influence on the mind.

BOTANICAL AND PHYTOCHEMICAL INFORMATION

There are twenty-eight known species of lavender, an evergreen, shrubby perennial. It has small, slender leaves, and its flowers are spikes of aromatic, two-lobed flowers that are usually purple or blue, but can vary from soft pink to bright pink. Depending on the species, it grows from eight to forty inches in height, and its leaves and bracts vary from a rich green to silver gray. Lavender flowers have a bittersweet smell, while its leaves have a balsamic scent.

The aromatic oil of lavender is extracted from the oil glands of the above-ground parts of the plant. The species known for the best-quality essential oil are *L. stoechas* and *L. angustifolia*. Up to 1.5 percent of the plant is composed of volatile oils that contain a variety of tannins, terpenes, and coumarins. Chemicals identified in lavender, including linalyl acetate, linalool, and lavendalol have have measurable calming effects in animals.

THE SCIENCE OF LAVENDER

Lavender oil has traditionally been used as an antiseptic, a mild sedative, and a painkiller. Modern studies have shown lavender to have an antiseptic effect on both bacteria and fungi.[1, 2] This property has been exploited to treat conditions ranging from wound infections to diaper rash. As a component of mouthwash, lavender may also reduce the chance for gum infections.

Midwives have extolled the virtues of lavender since the Middle Ages. It was burned in delivery rooms to reduce infections and used in sitz baths to soothe discomfort after delivery. Recent studies have suggested that lavender oil added to a bath may reduce some of a woman's discomfort after childbirth, providing tentative support for one of its traditional applications.[3]

Lavender is most widely recommended for its sedative properties. An Austrian study showed that lavender oil and two of its components had pro-

nounced tranquilizing effects in mice.[4] At sufficient concentrations, lavender was not only sedating in normal mice but had a substantial calming effect in animals that were previously given a stimulating dose of caffeine. A French report found that lavender oil was sedating, but that its efficacy diminished after five days.[5] An animal study from England showed that lavender was even able to reduce stress and travel sickness in pigs.[6]

Although lavender has been used to calm human minds for millennia, its sedating influence in people has not been well documented. Following the French penchant for fragrances, a study from Lyon, France, reported that people exposed to lavender oil had reductions in several physiological measures of stress.[7] In an English report, patients admitted to an intensive-care unit were studied to see if there were benefits of adding lavender oil to massage therapy. Although no objective differences were found between those that did and did not experience the aromatherapy, patients who were exposed to lavender reported less anxiety and a better mood.[8]

A novel use for lavender oil was recently described by a Scottish group of researchers who applied essential oils including lavender, thyme, rosemary, and cedarwood to the scalps of people with a condition known as alopecia areata. People with this problem, usually resulting from an autoimmune inflammatory process, lose patches of hair. This study, in which essential oils were massaged into patients' bald spots, reported improvement in over 40 percent of those receiving the essential oils, compared with only 15 percent treated with a non-herbalized carrier oil.[9]

THE PRACTICAL USE OF LAVENDER

In ancient herbal compendiums, lavender was reported to reduce the sting of insect bites, cool the pain of burns, soothe sore throats, relieve headaches, and calm stomach upsets. Applied to emotional concerns, lavender has a traditional role in the treatment of insomnia, anxiety, and melancholia. Water made from lavender flowers, applied as a skin toner, renews cells and treats acne. This multitalented plant can aid in digestive problems ranging from a gassy stomach to bad breath.

Lavender aromatherapy provides a subtle soothing influence. We regularly recommend adding drops of lavender fragrance to massage and facial oils to encourage relaxation. At the Chopra Center we apply eye packs and warmed shoulder pillows scented with lavender for relaxation before treatments.

Lavender is an important component of our sleep routine, in which we recommend a few drops of the essential oil added to a bath before bed. As a component of our prenatal program, new mothers are encouraged to take lavender sitz baths after giving birth, to soothe irritated tissues. Lavender tea is beneficial to calm mild anxiety.

HOW TO USE LAVENDER

As a tea for anxiety, tension headaches, and depression, steep two teaspoons of dried lavender flowers in one cup of boiling water. Add a few drops of lavender essential oil to a neutral massage oil and apply to the temples and nape of the neck for neck strain and headaches. A drop of the undiluted essential oil can be applied directly to insect bites and stings to relieve burning.

For mild digestive upsets, try adding a few drops of lavender oil to a sugar cube and allow it to slowly dissolve in your mouth. For irritated tissues or muscles, add five to ten drops to your bath water. As a sleeping aid, diffuse the essential oil in your bedroom, or keep a lavender flower sachet on your pillow. Children who are having trouble settling down to sleep often respond to this approach.

AYURVEDA AND LAVENDER

Although lavender was not known to the original Ayurvedic doctors, its herbal energetics can be understood in Ayurvedic terms. Its mildly pungent taste and slightly cooling influence make it a useful herb for all three mind-body constitutions. Lavender oil pacifies both Pitta and Kapha and has a balancing effect on Vata. It can calm an agitated mind without creating undue dullness.

PRECAUTIONS

Other than a rare skin sensitivity to the essential oil, this gentle plant has a high safety profile.

Circulatory/Respiratory	Detoxifier	Digestive	Immune Enhancer	Men's Health
		X		
Metabolic	Nervine	Rejuvenative	Rheumatic	Women's Health
	X			X

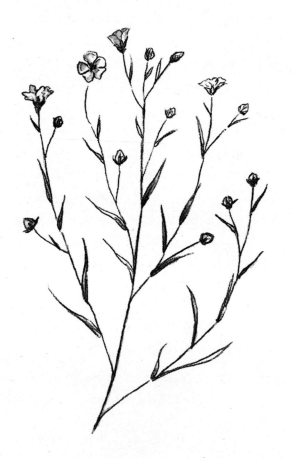

LINUM USITATISSIMUM

FAMILIAR: **flaxseed, linseed**
LATIN: *Linum usitatissimum*
SANSKRIT: uma

Flax has been part of the diets of human beings since the dawn of civilization. Archeologists have discovered irrigation systems in seven-thousand-year-old Mesopotamian cities that supported the cultivation of flax. Flax was one of the major sources of clothing fiber until the late eighteenth century, when cotton became popular. Native to the temperate regions of Asia and Europe, flax was introduced to North America in the early 1600s, and it flourished there. It is now grown throughout the world as a source of food, fiber, and oil.

Flaxseeds are a valuable health-promoting nutritional substance. In addition to providing a rich source of both soluble and insoluble fiber, flax supplies important omega-3 fatty acids and phyto-estrogens. In the Ayurvedic tradition, flax has been used in the treatment of respiratory disorders, digestive complaints, and urinary tract irritations. Hippocrates described the benefits of flaxseed in the treatment of abdominal cramping in the seventh century B.C.

BOTANICAL AND PHYTOCHEMICAL INFORMATION

Flax is an annual plant that grows two to four feet in height. It has a relatively thin stalk with elongated leaves and attractive blue or white flowers. Each small fruit yields ten yellowish to dark brown seeds, which are harvested in early autumn. The seeds are odorless, with an outer mucilaginous wall that swells when exposed to water.

Flaxseeds consist of 20 percent protein, 40 percent fat, and 28 percent fiber, with the remainder composed of water, vitamins, and minerals. Abundant in polyunsaturated fatty acids, flaxseeds are among the richest natural sources of alpha-linolenic acid (ALA), an omega-3 fatty acid that has been shown to help lower cholesterol levels and dampen inflammatory reactions.

THE SCIENCE OF FLAXSEED

Several studies have indicated a beneficial role for flaxseed on health. Adding flaxseed to the diet may help lower serum cholesterol levels in both animals and human beings. A recent study in rabbits showed that supplementing their diet with flaxseeds reduced the deposition of fat into major blood vessels by over two-thirds, even when the alpha-linolenic component was removed.[1] In another recent study involving rabbits, a phytoestrogen component of flaxseed, SDG, was found to reduce serum cholesterol, increase HDL cholesterol (the "good" cholesterol), and reduce the amount of atherosclerosis.[2]

Studies in people have also suggested some benefit from flaxseed in lowering cholesterol levels. In a Canadian study of people with high cholesterol levels given muffins with 50 grams of defatted flaxseed each day, there was a small but significant reduction in total and LDL cholesterol levels.[3] In another report of people consuming 50 grams of flaxseed daily, there was a reduction in their LDL cholesterol levels of 8 percent after only one month.[4] Although not every study has shown a definite benefit of flaxseed on cholesterol levels, most reports have suggested that flaxseed provides a safe and moderately effective way to lower one of the major risk factors for heart disease.

In addition to serving as a source of omega-3 fatty acids, flaxseed is the highest natural supplier of lignans, which are a type of phytoestrogen. Several studies in animals have suggested that the lignans in flaxseed have protective effects against hormonally sensitive tumors, particularly breast cancer, but also colon cancer and malignant melanoma.[5-7] Lignans are known to alter the metabolism of sex hormones, which may partially explain their beneficial role in cancer.[8] Although we do not yet know how and to what extent flaxseed can influence our susceptibility to cancer, there is convincing evidence in human beings that adding flaxseed to the diet has potentially important effects on hormone levels.[9]

A potentially useful role for flaxseed is in the treatment of inflammatory conditions. In animal studies, the high concentration of omega-3 fatty acids in flaxseed has been shown to reduce inflammatory prostaglandins. This property has been tested in people in two autoimmune inflammatory conditions: rheumatoid arthritis (RA) and systemic lupus erythematosis (SLE). In a report from Finland of twenty-two patients with RA, the addition of flaxseed to their diet did not prove beneficial in reducing their symptoms.[10] In a Canadian study of nine people with inflammatory problems in their kidneys resulting from SLE, flaxseed resulted in many positive changes, including improvements in kidney function, a reduction in inflammatory chemicals in the blood, and lower cholesterol levels.[11] Clearly, further research is indicated to assess the potential role of flaxseed in combating inflammatory and autoimmune disorders.

THE PRACTICAL USE OF FLAXSEED

Adding flaxseed to your diet is one of the easiest and least expensive ways to enhance your health. In addition to the potential benefits of flaxseed in reducing your risk for cardiovascular disease and cancer, flaxseed is an excellent source of fiber that improves bowel function.[12] You can use whole flaxseeds, or grind them in a coffee grinder. Flaxseed can be added to granola, sprinkled on sautéed vegetables or combined with wheat flour for breads and muffins. Whole flaxseed can be stored at room temperature for up to a year. Milled flaxseed should be refrigerated once ground and used within one month.

Several farms and dairies are adding flaxseed to the feed of chickens and cows in order to increase the amount of omega-3 fatty acids in eggs and milk. It will be interesting to see if these food products can help lower cholesterol levels.

Traditionally, flaxseed has been used as a poultice for skin infections and abscesses. A few tablespoonfuls are wrapped in a white cotton bandage and boiled in water until the seeds are soft. They are then applied to the wound and covered for fifteen minutes every few hours. The flaxseed has a drawing effect and maintains heat in the area to increase circulation.

HOW TO USE FLAXSEED

Flaxseeds are readily available in health-food stores and many grocery stores. The usual dosage in studies that have shown a benefit from the addition of flaxseed is 50 grams per day, providing about 6 grams of dietary fiber. Fifty grams is equivalent to about one-quarter cup of flaxseeds daily. Use flaxseeds liberally in your cooking and baking, and your body will benefit.

AYURVEDA AND FLAXSEED

According to Ayurveda, raw flaxseeds are soothing and emollient, whereas roasted seeds have a drier, hotter quality. Flaxseeds carry the primary tastes of sweet and astringent, with a heating potency. They are pacifying to Vata, but may be mildly aggravating to Pitta and Kapha when taken in high dosages.

PRECAUTIONS

As a component of human diets for thousands of years, flaxseed is a very safe nutritional product. Respiratory allergies have been reported in textile workers who inhale the fibers of flax, but this is not relevant to the internal ingestion of the seeds. Flaxseed acts as a mild bulk laxative, similar to psyllium. It is more appropriately used as a preventive bowel tonic than for the acute treatment of constipation.

Circulatory/Respiratory	Detoxifier	Digestive	Immune Enhancer	Men's Health
X		X		
Metabolic	Nervine	Rejuvenative	Rheumatic	Women's Health
			X	

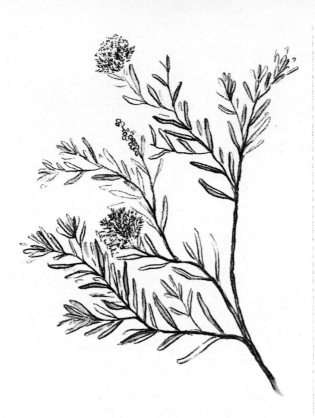

MELALEUCA
ALTERNIFOLIA

FAMILIAR: **tea tree**
LATIN: *Melaleuca alternifolia*

The tea tree has been valued by Australian Aborigines since before recorded history. Its name is attributed to the eighteenth-century English explorer Captain James Cook, who added the leaves of the tree to an herbal brew in order to make his crew's beer more palatable. A century and a half later, an Australian surgeon described the use of tea tree oil as an antiseptic to reduce surgical infections. A resurgence of interest in tea tree has been fueled by studies over the past ten years, which have confirmed its value as an effective and safe natural germicidal agent in a wide range of conditions from acne to athlete's foot.

BOTANICAL AND PHYTOCHEMICAL INFORMATION

There are over three hundred members of the melaleuca family, but it is *Melaleuca alternifolia* that has risen to prominence for its beneficial essential oil. A rapidly growing evergreen tree that reaches twenty-five feet in height, it has a soft, papery bark with clusters of small white flowers. Native to southeast Australia, tea trees are now grown commercially in Africa, Central America, and India.

The essential oil of tea tree is obtained from the leaves through steam distillation. It contains a number of terpenes, of which terpinen-4-ol is believed to be responsible for its beneficial anti-infective activity. Other volatile constituents, including limonene, alpha-terpinen, cineole, and aromadendrene, are present in lower concentrations and appear responsible for the occasional skin irritations that are reported by people sensitive to tea tree oil. Trees that produce high levels of terpinen-4-ol are being propagated in order to maximize the therapeutic-to-toxic ratio of essential oil components.[1]

THE SCIENCE OF
TEA TREE OIL

Tea tree oil first played an important role in Western society during World War II, when it was added to machinery oil for equipment used in weapons production. The antibiotic properties of tea tree were said to reduce the infections in factory workers who injured their hands on the munitions production line. The commercial development of Australian tea tree farms in the early 1980s stimulated scientific research into its therapeutic effects. Many studies published within the past decade have documented unique beneficial qualities of tea tree oil.

Tea tree has demonstrated value in the treatment of fungal skin infections. A study evaluating the benefit of a 10-percent tea tree oil cream applied to people with athlete's foot caused by the fungus *Tinea pedis* showed that the cream resulted in clinical improvement in over 60 percent of people, and the fungus was completely eliminated in about 30 percent.[2] A study from New York looked at the role of tea tree in the treatment of the most common nail fungus called onychomycosis and found that tea tree oil was as effective as the most popular pharmaceutical medicine.[3] Laboratory studies looking at tea tree oil's potency against a wide range of potential disease-causing fungal organisms have shown it to be efficacious at concen-

trations readily achieved by applying the oil to the skin.[4]

Tea tree oil has been consistently effective against different species of candida. This ubiquitous yeast can cause both vaginal and oral infections, and is capable of invading deeper tissues if a person's immune system is compromised. Studies from the Netherlands have demonstrated that tea tree oil is active against most species of candida, even after it has been diluted in a suppository.[5] As a component of a mouthwash, it may be helpful in the treatment of oral candida infections.

Tea tree oil is also effective against a wide range of bacteria. It has been studied as a potential antimicrobial agent in the treatment of skin infections and has been found active against many potentially harmful bacteria. Tea tree oil seems to have a selective effect against potentially harmful bacteria while only minimally interfering with the normal bacteria that usually inhabit our skin.[6] It is active against the germs that cause acne and has been shown to be as effective as the most commonly used topical acne medication, benzoyl peroxide.[7, 8] Although tea tree takes somewhat longer to act, it has fewer negative side effects.

Tea tree oil has been studied in the treatment of burns. It is effective in reducing some of the common infections encountered in burn units, but other potentially serious germs are not sensitive to tea tree oil.[9]

Therefore it is not recommended for patients with severe scaldings, but may still have value in the treatment of minor burn injuries.

A potentially important use for tea tree oil is in reducing the spread of methicillin-resistant staphylococcus infections (MRSAs). This virulent bacteria is commonly found in hospitals and nursing homes, where it is often spread by staff members. In an Australian study, all sixty-six samples of MRSA were sensitive to tea tree oil at relatively low concentrations. Adding tea tree oil to hand-washing lotions may provide a safe and effective alternative to the chemical antibacterial soaps currently in widespread use.[10]

THE PRACTICAL USE OF TEA TREE OIL

Tea tree oil is finding its way into an expanding range of health-care products. As an essential oil, it can be applied directly to fungal skin infections such as athlete's foot. Most people tolerate the direct application of pure tea tree oil, although occasionally it results in a skin reaction requiring its discontinuation. The oil can also be directly applied to acne sores, but again, if irritation develops, it should be stopped. As a component of a lotion or cream, tea tree oil can be applied to minor cuts, abrasions, and burns.

Tea tree oil is showing up in toothpaste and mouthwash. You can make your own

solution by adding drops of tea tree oil to water for use as a mouthwash or throat gargle. Deodorants, shampoos, throat lozenges, soaps, and even animal-care products with tea tree oil are now being sold in the marketplace. Capitalizing on its potency against candida, douches and suppositories containing tea tree oil are potentially useful for the treatment of vaginal yeast infections. Tea tree is active against another common vaginal infectious agent, trichomonas. A study from the 1960s suggested that a vaginal douche with tea tree oil could be useful in the treatment of cervical and vaginal infections, but needed to be applied weekly for four to six weeks.[11] Tea tree oil vaginal suppositories are currently available and may be effective, but can occasionally cause vaginal irritation that may be difficult to distinguish from the symptoms of the original infection.[12] If itching and a discharge persist after five days, the tea tree product should be discontinued and medical advice sought.

HOW TO USE TEA TREE OIL

Every household should keep some tea tree oil close at hand. It can be applied directly to skin irritations, or diluted into a bland cream or lotion. It mixes well with a vitamin E cream or aloe vera gel for minor abrasions and burns. Add ten drops of tea tree oil to four ounces of warm water, and use as a gargle or mouthwash. If you are using tea tree oil in the treatment of athlete's foot or other minor fungal infections, apply it twice daily and observe the problem area to see if there is improvement after several days of usage. For stubborn fungal infections, application of tea tree oil may be necessary for months until the problem is resolved. Commercially available skin creams containing tea tree can be useful to treat and prevent diaper rash, but watch your baby's skin closely to ensure that he or she is not developing a negative reaction.

AYURVEDA AND TEA TREE OIL

From an Ayurvedic perspective, tea tree oil carries the bitter, pungent, astringent, and sweet tastes. It cools the inflammation of Pitta, clears the congestion of Kapha, and is essentially neutral toward Vata. Tea tree oil has a net cooling influence on the system.

PRECAUTIONS

Up to ten percent of people may have a skin sensitivity to tea tree oil.[13] Although the chemical constituent cineole is usually held responsible, several other components can also be irritating in susceptible people.[14] A tea made from the leaves of the tea tree is commonly used by Aboriginal natives, but generally should be avoided due to concerns about toxicity. A case has been reported of accidental poisoning in a two-year-old boy who ingested two teaspoons of tea tree oil. The symptoms were mental confusion and unsteadiness that resolved after five hours.[15]

Circulatory/Respiratory	Detoxifier	Digestive	Immune Enhancer	Men's Health
	X			
Metabolic	Nervine	Rejuvenative	Rheumatic	Women's Health
			X	

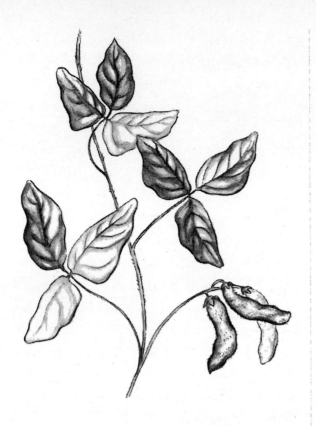

MUCUNA
PRURIENS

FAMILIAR: **atmagupta, cowage,
cowitch plant**
LATIN: *Mucuna pruriens*
SANSKRIT: atmagupta, kapikacchu,
vanari

The ancient Ayurvedic physician Sushruta described atmagupta as one of the premiere rejuvenative substances for both men and women. It has been considered a powerful aphrodisiac for thousands of years, which, according to Ayurveda, implies enhancing both sexual potency and fertility. Atmagupta is held in high esteem as a tonic herb to reverse the aging process. Modern studies have demonstrated a therapeutic role for it in the treatment of Parkinson's disease and diabetes, which may partially explain its reputation as a vitality-restoring herb.

As a member of the legume family, atmagupta is a nutritionally rich substance containing over 25 percent protein.[1] It is also a rich source of complex carbohydrates and fiber. It contains many unique alkaloids that have received only preliminary scientific investigation. The efficacy of atmagupta in the treatment of Parkinson's disease is due in part to its ability to generate L-dopa (L-dihydroxyphenylalanine) from simpler amino acids. The pharmacological mechanisms of its other demonstrated medicinal properties, from lowering blood sugar to treating snakebite, remain to be elucidated.

BOTANICAL AND PHOTOCHEMICAL INFORMATION

Mucuna pruriens is a climbing legume that thrives in tropical climates. It grows wild in India and the Caribbean, and has been identified in southern Florida. The name *pruriens* (from the Latin *prurire,* to itch) refers to the irritation caused by tiny barbs on its pods that attach to the skin of unsuspecting harvesters. Ayurvedic doctors use the processed pods to treat internal parasites, but it is the inner seed that is the primary medicinal product.

The plant is an annual climber with slender vines and clusters of three leaves. It produces inch-and-a-half-wide flowers that yield the two- to three-inch-long curved pods containing the dark seeds. Several unique alkaloids, including mucunine, mucunadine, prurienine, and prurieninine, have been identified in atmagupta, as well as a variety of organic acids, sterols, tannins, and L-dopa and other amino acids. The complex sugars of atmagupta are broken down with boiling, but the L-dopa content is not substantially affected.[2]

THE SCIENCE OF ATMAGUPTA

Although atmagupta has been traditionally extolled as a rejuvenative substance, scientific investigation into this tonic herb has been in two main areas, the treatment of Parkinson's disease and the treatment of diabetes mellitus. Although Parkinson's disease was first described in the West by James Parkinson in the early nineteenth century, a neurological condition that included tremor, slow movements, and muscle stiffness was known to ancient Ayurvedic doctors as Kampavata.[3] We now attribute this disabling degenerative condition to diminishing amounts of the natural brain chemical dopamine. The most effective modern treatment for this illness is to enhance the production of dopamine by providing its precursor chemical, L-dopa, which is converted in the brain to dopamine. Atmagupta has the natural ability to generate L-dopa in concentrations up to 6 percent of its dry weight when grown under ideal conditions.[4] A recent scientific study of sixty patients with Parkinson's disease found that those taking atmagupta showed substantial reductions in their symptoms and improvement in their overall quality of life within twelve weeks of treatment.[5] This confirmed an earlier report of twenty-three patients given atmagupta who demonstrated benefits in every aspect of the illness, including reduction in muscle stiffness and tremors, along with improvements in walking, dressing, and speech function.[6] An interesting aspect of this study was the recognition that the calculated dose of L-dopa was generally lower than is usually required to see a therapeutic effect, and conventional side effects were noticeably absent. These observations suggest that other unidentified constituents of atmagupta may have therapeutic value and help to counteract the side effects of the "active" chemicals.

Atmagupta has also shown potential medicinal benefit in the treatment of diabetes mellitus. Diabetic rabbits given atmagupta had significant reductions in their blood sugar levels.[7] A study published over thirty years ago in rats found that atmagupta reduced both blood glucose and cholesterol levels.[8] Although *Mucuna pruriens* has been used classically to stabilize metabolic function in people, scientific research has not yet been focused on its value in the treatment of diabetes in human beings.

An interesting study reported from London looked at the effects of *Mucuna pruriens* on the treatment of snakebite. Although, fortunately, this is not a common concern in most Western countries, it is a recurring health problem in many tropical regions of the world. Some snake venoms act by causing the blood to clot, and effective herbal approaches, including atmagupta, have been shown to act by inhibiting the clotting cascade.[9] The potential benefit of atmagupta on a whole range of clotting disorders remains to be explored.

Science has just scratched the surface of the therapeutic potential of atmagupta. Its role in the treatment of impotency and infertility is an area of great potential value, and its traditional use as a rejuvenative substance is worthy of serious scientific evaluation.

THE PRACTICAL USE OF ATMAGUPTA

Atmagupta is traditionally used as a tonic for men and women in conditions of low energy and reduced sexual desire or potency. A teaspoon of the powdered seeds is mixed in sweetened warm milk. It is a common component of Ayurvedic rejuvenative formulas that include ashwagandha, shatavari, or amalaki. It can be taken on a daily basis or prior to an anticipated intimate encounter.

Studies using atmagupta for Parkinson's disease have used starting doses of approximately 5 grams, gradually increasing the amount as needed. If you have Parkinson's disease, discuss the use of atmagupta with your health-care provider before using it. The interaction of atmagupta with standard Parkinson's disease medications has not been studied, and therefore adding this herbal medicine should only be done under close medical supervision. Atmagupta is used in lower doses as a rejuvenating substance and has a long-established traditional history of safety.

HOW TO USE ATMAGUPTA

Atmagupta is not yet readily available in the West, although it is finding its way into more Ayurvedic herbal mixtures. It is usually combined with ashwagandha as part of a male potency formula, where it is present in doses of 100 to 200 milligrams. Powdered atmagupta is also available from a few herbal importers. The suggested dose to enhance vitality is 1 teaspoon daily, mixed in warm milk.

AYURVEDA AND ATMAGUPTA

Atmagupta carries the sweet and bitter tastes. It has a warming effect on the physiology and is useful in balancing all three doshas. In excess, it can increase Kapha and Pitta. It is a valuable Vata balancing tonic.

PRECAUTIONS

The pods of *Mucuna pruriens* can cause pronounced itching. In a 1985 case, a Hispanic New Jersey couple developed an irritating rash as a result of exposure to what they called "voodoo beans."[10] The emergency medical technician and the emergency room nurse who treated them developed the same skin irritation. The beans were later identified as *Mucuna pruriens*. The inner seeds, which are used medicinally, do not have an irritating effect.

An outbreak of toxic psychosis was reported from Mozambique in 1990.[11] During a time of severe famine, residents of a rural district developed headache and confusion, attributed to the consumption of excessive amounts of *Mucuna pruriens* seeds as a source of nourishment. Because of a water shortage, the seeds were not properly cooked, which contributed to the toxic effects.

Although these rare complications are interesting, they are clearly extreme and not relevant to the usual therapeutic use of atmagupta, which has a high safety profile as a rejuvenative tonic. Caution should be exercised if you are taking it with any other medications that may act upon the nervous system.

Circulatory/Respiratory	Detoxifier	Digestive	Immune Enhancer	Men's Health
				X
Metabolic	Nervine	Rejuvenative	Rheumatic	Women's Health
	X	X		

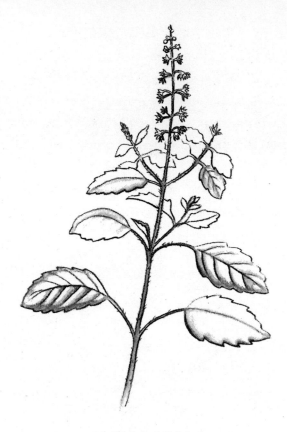

OCIMUM SANCTUM

FAMILIAR: **holy basil, sacred basil**
LATIN: *Ocimum sanctum*
SANSKRIT: Tulsi, Tulasi

Holy basil has both medicinal and spiritual significance in Ayurveda. It is sacred to Lord Vishnu, the Hindu god of preservation, and is considered purifying to body, mind, and spirit. A living tulsi plant is kept in many Indian homes, where it is endowed with a sacred aura and believed to provide divine protection for the household. Rosaries made from its cut stems are commonly used as meditation beads.

Closely related to the sweet basil plant widely available in the West, holy basil has been used as a valued culinary and medicinal herb. Its traditional use has been in the treatment of colds and flus, where its purifying actions are believed to cleanse the respiratory tract of toxins. It is also helpful in the relief of digestive gas and bloating. Recent scientific reports have confirmed the healing properties of holy basil in medical conditions ranging from diabetes to cancer.

BOTANICAL AND PHYTOCHEMICAL INFORMATION

Basil is found on almost every continent, although *Ocimum sanctum* is native to the Indian subcontinent. It grows to about eighteen inches in height, with oval serrated leaves and delicate lavender-colored flowers. The plant is an annual in the wild but can be maintained as a perennial by trimming it before it is allowed to form seeds. The fruit consists of tiny rust-colored nuts.

The leaves are the richest source of essential oil, which contains eugenol, nerol, camphor, and a variety of terpenes and flavonoids. A recent analysis of holy basil oil revealed five fatty acids, including stearic, palmitic, oleic, linoleic, and linolenic. The triglyceride component was found to have potent anti-inflammatory properties. The oil is antiseptic against a wide range of disease-causing organisms including bacteria, fungi, and parasites. Both water- and alcohol-based extracts of basil leaves have demonstrated pharmacological activity.

THE SCIENCE OF TULSI

Holy basil oil has antioxidant and anti-inflammatory activity. Several studies have demonstrated that constituents of holy basil can neutralize free radicals and inhibit the production of inflammatory prostaglandins.[1, 2] An animal study found an extract of holy basil to be essentially equivalent to a standard dose of aspirin.[3] These effects may explain one of tulsi's traditional roles in the treatment of pain and arthritis.

The antioxidant properties of holy basil may also underlie its effectiveness in dampening the effects of stress on the physiology. A study in rats subjected to restraint stress found that those taking holy basil had less derangement in their biochemistry than did animals receiving a placebo.[4] In addition to its ability to dampen the chemical changes of stress, holy basil also appears to influence the neurochemistry of the brain in a manner similar to antidepressant medications.[5] Holy basil has even been shown to reduce the levels of stress hormones produced when an animal is subjected to chronic noise stress.[6]

These interesting pharmacological properties have recently been applied to different clinical situations with potentially important results. A number of studies have looked at the ability of holy basil to protect healthy cells from the toxicity associated with radiation and chemotherapy for cancer.[7, 8] Components of holy basil consistently limited the damage that radiation causes to the bone marrow and digestive tract in animals. When the cells were looked at microscopically, those animals that received holy basil had less chromosomal damage than those that received a placebo.[9]

Holy basil has also been shown to protect the heart from damage caused by a widely used chemotherapy drug, adriamycin.[10] It seems to work by protecting components of heart and liver cells from oxidative damage caused by free radicals generated by the chemotherapy. Other studies have shown holy basil to have a protective effect against chemical carcinogens.[11, 12] Adding to its potential value in the prevention and treatment of cancer, holy basil has also been shown to enhance different aspects of the immune response in animals.[13]

Another medical condition that holy basil may benefit is diabetes. Animal studies have shown holy basil to have substantial blood-sugar-lowering effects, similar to standard oral diabetes medications.[14, 15] It also appears capable of lowering cholesterol and triglyceride levels.[16] Diabetes is one of the few areas where holy basil has been formally tested in people. In a recent study of forty patients with non-insulin-dependent diabetes mellitus (NIDDM), people taking 2.5 grams of dried tulsi leaf powder every morning showed significant reductions in their blood glucose levels first thing in the morning as well as after their meals.[17] In addition to lower glucose levels, they also had a mild reduction in their cholesterol levels. This simple intervention could have a substantial impact on this common health problem, particularly in regions where expensive diabetes medication is out of reach for many people.

One of tulsi's traditional uses has been in the treatment of digestive disorders ranging from heartburn to bloating. Studies in animals have suggested that there is a scientific basis to these long-standing claims. Holy basil has been shown to have significant anti-ulcer activity.[18] It reduces the effect of peptic acid or irritating drugs on the stomach lining and increases the production of protective stomach mucus.[19]

This popular plant has many potential therapeutic applications. In addition to the uses reviewed above, tulsi may possess useful antibiotic activity, have a blood-pressure-lowering effect, and be effective as a birth-control agent. This sacred healing plant deserves further scientific attention.

THE PRACTICAL USE OF HOLY BASIL

Tulsi leaves are traditionally used to make a strong tea for the treatment of colds, flus, and sore throats. Fresh, dried, or powdered leaves are taken after meals to soothe digestive upset. The extract can be applied directly to acne lesions, where its antibiotic effect hastens healing. The juice of the fresh leaves can also be applied topically to skin conditions ranging from allergic rashes to athlete's foot.

If you are taking holy basil for its stress-relieving properties, I recommend you obtain seeds or cuttings and grow your own plant. Place the seeds between warm, moist paper towels for a day and then bury them a half-inch under the surface in rich potting soil. A sprout will break through within ten days. Once it reaches about a foot in height, pinch back any flowers to keep it from going to seed, or allow it to seed and start a new generation. Nibble on a few leaves every day for their health-promoting effects.

HOW TO USE HOLY BASIL

Most Indian food stores carry tulsi leaves in a dried or powdered form. If you are taking holy basil for a specific health concern, such as diabetes or indigestion, take a standard dose of one-half teaspoon three times daily after meals. If you are using it as a nutritional aid while undergoing chemotherapy, prepare a strong holy basil tea by placing one tablespoon of dried leaves per pint of hot water and sipping it throughout the day, aiming to drink two to four pints within twenty-four hours. If you are inspired to grow your own plant, use holy basil freely in your cooking as well as in the making of freshly brewed tea.

If you cannot find holy basil *(Ocimum sanctum)*, common sweet basil *(Ocimum basilicum)* is a reasonable substitute. Although not as extensively studied as holy basil, sweet basil does appear to share many of the same phytochemical and medicinal properties.

TULSI AND AYURVEDA

According to Ayurveda, Tulsi creates purity and lightness in the body. It carries the bitter, pungent, and astringent tastes, and generates a warming influence on the physiology. It has a sweet post-digestive effect. Its effect on the doshas is predominantly Kapha-reducing, but it can be used to pacify Vata and Pitta as well. In severely overheated individuals, Tulsi can have a mildly Pitta-aggravating effect.

PRECAUTIONS

Holy basil is generally a very safe healing herb. Studies from the 1970s suggested that holy basil might have a mild anti-fertility effect in animals. Although this has not been shown to occur in people, if you are pregnant or trying to become pregnant, do not take medicinal doses of holy basil.

Circulatory/Respiratory	Detoxifier	Digestive	Immune Enhancer	Men's Health
X		X	X	
Metabolic	Nervine	Rejuvenative	Rheumatic	Women's Health
X				

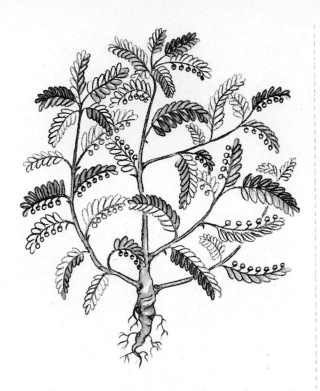

PHYLLANTHUS
NIRURI

FAMILIAR: **phyllanthus**

LATIN: *Phyllanthus niruri, Phyllanthus amanus*

SANSKRIT: bhumyaamalaki, bahupatra

Known for thousands of years to Ayurvedic doctors, phyllanthus has been respected as a detoxifing herb throughout Asia, Africa, and Latin America. It has been used in conditions ranging from recurrent fevers to skin disorders to hiccups. Ayurvedic physicians recognized the ability of phyllanthus to reduce the jaundice associated with liver ailments. Recent scientific investigations have supported the role of phyllanthus as a liver protectant, particularly in response to the hepatitis B virus.

BOTANICAL AND PHYTOCHEMICAL INFORMATION

Phyllanthus niruri is a small branching annual plant that is one and one-half to two feet in height at maturity. It has many small leaves with very small flowers. The young leaves are used for infectious and inflammatory conditions, while the juice of the leaves is applied to irritated skin lesions. The leaves, stems, flowers, and roots all have medicinal value.

Several unique chemical constituents have been characterized in phyllanthus. Lignans called phyllanthum and hypophyllanthum have been identified in the leaves. Organic acids and alkaloids have been found in the leaves and roots. Extracts of phyllanthus have been demonstrated to inhibit the replication of viral DNA, block the transmission of pain impulses, reduce muscle spasms, and lower blood sugar, but the precise chemicals responsible for these specific effects remain to be fully defined.

THE SCIENCE OF PHYLLANTHUS

Dozens of scientific studies have been published on phyllanthus over the past fifteen years. Most research has focused on the ability of chemicals in phyllanthus to bind to various components of the hepatitis B virus. Early studies in mice suggested that extracts of phyllanthus could eliminate the markers of viral infection in a high percentage of animals.[1] These encouraging laboratory results were subsequently applied to people who were carriers of the hepatitis B virus. In a study from India, almost 60 percent of people with hepatitis B showed conversion of their blood tests from positive to negative.[2] Further studies clarified the role of phyllanthus as binding to proteins produced by the virus and reducing the activity of viral DNA.[3, 4]

Many studies, but not every one, have shown positive results. A report from Thailand found that only 5 to 6 percent of adults carrying hepatitis B virus showed conversion of their blood tests from positive to negative.[5] A Bombay study of thirty chronic carriers of hepatitis failed to find any clearing of the markers for hepatitis after one to two months of treatment with phyllanthus.[6] These contradictory findings highlight the fact that science rarely moves in a straight line. However, in view of the limited treatment options available to people with chronic hepatitis, phyllanthus is a potential bright spot on the therapeutic horizon.

Phyllanthus has also shown potential in the treatment of other viral infections. Constituents of phyllanthus have demonstrated activity against the Epstein-Barr virus, the infectious agent responsible for mononucleosis and loosely associated with chronic fatigue syndrome.[7] Other researchers have suggested that phyllanthus may be active against the HIV virus responsible for AIDS. A report from Japan found that an extract of phyllanthus could inhibit the enzyme that enables HIV to reproduce itself.[8] These preliminary laboratory findings are encouraging, but we have some distance to go before they can be systematically applied to people with AIDS.

Phyllanthus also shows promise in protecting the liver from other toxic insults. A recent report found that it reduced the damage to liver enzymes caused by excessive alcohol.[9] Another study demonstrated the ability of phyllanthus to reduce the liver damage caused by toxic chemicals, including carbon tetrachloride and galactosamine.[10] How phyllanthus protects the liver remains to be discovered, but it seems that this ancient healing plant contains potential healing treasures.

In addition to its value in liver conditions, phyllanthus has been studied for its possible therapeutic role in several other medical conditions. In both India and Latin America, it is a popular remedy for kidney stones. Researchers in Brazil have studied the effects of phyllanthus on the urinary system and have made some interesting discoveries. In one report it was found to reduce the likelihood of the smooth muscle lining of the urinary tract to go into spasm.[11] This relaxation effect could improve the ease with which small kidney stones are passed. In a recent report, phyllanthus was found to inhibit the formation of calcium oxalate crystals in kidney cells.[12] Phyllanthus has also shown promise in the treatment of high blood pressure, possibly by helping the kidney eliminate excess sodium from the body.[13] This same report also found that phyllanthus had a blood-sugar-lowering effect. These many beneficial properties of phyllanthus may help explain its traditional reputation as a therapeutic herb for kidney problems.

Finally, there have been several reports emphasizing the pain-relieving properties of phyllanthus. Its chemical constituents reduce both inflammatory and pain responses in animals through mechanisms that have not yet been determined.[14, 15] These properties, possibly reflecting interactions with the prostaglandin system, may ultimately account for the traditional role of phyllanthus in the treatment of chronic fevers and inflammatory conditions.

THE PRACTICAL USE OF PHYLLANTHUS

According to the Ayurvedic framework, the bitter detoxifying qualities of phyllanthus predict its therapeutic value in conditions characterized by excessive heat and toxicity. Since the liver is the primary organ of detoxification, liver ailments, including hepatitis, have traditionally been treated with phyllanthus. Almost all of the modern scientific studies on hepatitis have focused on hepatitis B. We do not yet know if phyllanthus has any beneficial role in the treatment of hepatitis A or C. It does seem to be quite safe, without reported side effects. If you are facing a liver problem for which you are considering using phyllanthus, we strongly encourage you discuss it with your health-care provider and establish objective ways to measure the presence or absence of a therapeutic effect. Most published studies have found that if phyllanthus is to show a benefit on blood markers of hepatitis, it will occur within the first two months of use. If no measurable effect is seen within this time frame, there is little justification in continuing it.

HOW TO USE PHYLLANTHUS

Phyllanthus is not widely known in the West. It is a component of several Ayurvedic liver formulas, where it is often combined with kutki. Phyllanthus is now available from several herb companies as a single herb, standardized to 10 milligrams of total sesquiterpenes. The usual dose of the nonprocessed herb is 250 to 500 milligrams, two to three times per day. The general recommendation is to use phyllanthus for up to two months at a time.

AYURVEDA AND PHYLLANTHUS

Phyllanthus is composed of the bitter, astringent, and sweet tastes. These are the three flavors that pacify Pitta. Because the bitter taste is predominant, phyllanthus also pacifies Kapha. It can be mildly aggravating to Vata. Its net effect is to have a cooling influence on the physiology.

PRECAUTIONS

No serious side effects have been reported with phyllanthus. Because of its cooling, detoxifying influence, it should be used cautiously by people who are depleted. If you are using phyllanthus with the specific intention of treating a viral illness, please work closely with your health-care provider to monitor its safety and efficacy.

Circulatory/Respiratory	Detoxifier	Digestive	Immune Enhancer	Men's Health
	X			
Metabolic	Nervine	Rejuvenative	Rheumatic	Women's Health

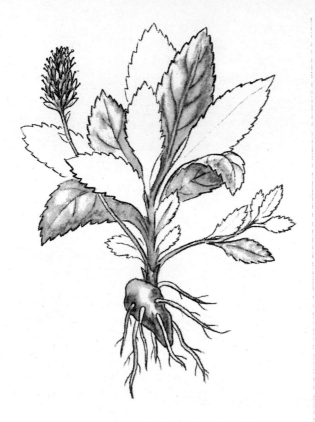

PICRORHIZA
KURROA

FAMILIAR: **kutki, picroliv**
LATIN: *Picrorhiza kurroa*
SANSKRIT: kutki, katuka

Although not yet well known in the West, kutki has a long-established reputation in Ayurveda as a detoxifier and liver tonic. This hardy, mountain-dwelling plant can be found above ten thousand feet in the Himalayan Mountains. The kutki plant produces pink flowers during the months of summer when the snow melts, but it is the underground roots and rhizomes that are harvested for their medicinal effects. Although used for thousands of years by Ayurvedic doctors, it has only recently received serious scientific attention for its liver-protecting properties. As chronic viral liver infections pose a growing public health threat in the West, botanical allies such as kutki may play an increasingly important role.

BOTANICAL AND PHYTOCHEMICAL INFORMATION

Kutki is a perennial shrub that has two- to four-inch leaves, small flowers, and a five- to ten-inch-long main root, from which the medicinal herb is obtained. It grows at high altitude in the northwestern Himalayas in the region of Kashmir. Close botanical relatives to kutki are found in Mongolia and Tibet.

Many different chemical constituents are found in the roots of kutki, including glucosides, flavonoids, and sterols. The component that has received the most attention is kutkin, which is a combination of two glucosides called glucoside-A and kutkoside. The most commonly available form of kutki is standardized to contain 10 milligrams of kutkin per tablet.

THE SCIENCE OF KUTKI

Exploring the traditional use of kutki in the treatment of bilious fever, studies from the mid-1960s reported that patients with infective hepatitis given kutki showed faster recoveries.[1] Many reports over the past ten years have confirmed the benefits of kutki in protecting the liver from a wide range of toxic and infectious insults. Investigation in animals has shown that kutki can help reverse the liver damage caused by poisonous mushrooms, noxious chemicals, and toxic amino acids.[2–4]

Although liver cancer is relatively rare in the West, it is one of the most common malignancies in developing countries. The major risk factors for liver cancer are hepatitis B viral infection and exposure to a food contaminant called aflatoxin. This toxic chemical, produced by a common mold, is a widespread problem throughout Africa and Asia. Animal studies from India have demonstrated that kutki protects the liver from most of the harmful effects of aflatoxin.[5] Kutki has also been shown to protect the liver against various tropical parasites and to strengthen the immune system's response to tuberculosis.[6, 7]

These infectious diseases and poisonings are fortunately uncommon in the West, but kutki may also provide benefit in two common conditions that affect the liver: alcoholism and hepatitis B. Animals exposed to enough alcohol to cause liver damage showed much less toxicity when they were also given kutki.[8] Another report from India demonstrated that in the laboratory kutki has some potential to neutralize components of the hepatitis B virus.[9] It also stimulates the flow of bile, which may be helpful in the prevention of gallstones.[10] The application of kutki's liver-protecting qualities to diseases in people still requires further research, but this herb seems to have considerable therapeutic potential. In some studies kutki is more potent than silybum, a popular herb that is commonly recommended for liver ailments.[11]

In addition to its potential role in the therapy of liver disease, kutki has been studied as a possible medicinal herb in the treatment of asthma and allergies. Laboratory studies have suggested that kutki dampens the release of allergy-causing chemicals and reduces the severity of airway spasm in animals.[12, 13] Chemical constituents of kutki also have anti-inflammatory activity and inhibit the action of histamine.[14, 15] Despite its suppression of an allergic response, kutki has been found to have immune-enhancing properties.[16] These combined effects give credence to the traditional use of kutki in the treatment of bronchial asthma and support the value of further scientific research on this ancient healing herb.

THE PRACTICAL USE OF KUTKI

Kutki is one of Ayurveda's powerful purifying herbs. Since the liver is the body's primary site of detoxification, kutki was classically used when congestion in the liver was identified. Kutki is now recommended when there is a challenge to the liver from toxins or infection. If someone has been abusing alcohol or drugs, or eating poorly, kutki can be a helpful component of a detoxification program. Although its role in the treatment of chronic hepatitis is receiving increasing attention, its clinical efficacy is yet to be determined. If you are facing a diagnosed liver problem such as chronic hepatitis, discuss the use of kutki with your health-care provider before using it.

Kutki also has a traditional role in the treatment of bronchitis and asthma. Its pungent bitterness is cleansing to the respiratory tract. It also has a mildly cathartic effect on the digestive system when taken in higher doses. Combined with amalaki and licorice, it can help relieve indigestion.

How to Use Kutki

Kutki is now available through major American herbal suppliers, where it goes by the name of picroliv. The usual dose is 300 milligrams two to three times daily. Take it for one month at a time, and assess whether it is achieving the effects you are seeking. Do not take it for longer than three months at a stretch.

Kutki is also a component of other herbal formulas for the liver, combined with other Ayurvedic or Western herbs. It combines well with turmeric, gotu kola, neem, and phyllanthus. A formulation combining kutki with silybum is currently available in the United States.

Ayurveda and Kutki

The predominant taste of kutki is bitter, with a secondary pungent component. It has a net cooling influence on the mind-body physiology. Kutki is most appropriate for Pitta and Kapha conditions. Its sustained use may be mildly Vata-aggravating. As a bitter detoxifying herb, it was traditionally recommended for toxic conditions of the blood, characterized by low-grade fevers, generalized pain, and fatigue.

Precautions

There are no reported cases of toxicity due to kutki. Because it has a strong detoxifying effect on the physiology, it should be used cautiously in people who have illnesses that are depleting. It is to be avoided during pregnancy. Although it has traditionally been used for lactating mothers to purify their milk, there are no scientific studies to verify its safety in young children; therefore, breastfeeding mothers should avoid it. If you have a form of chronic hepatitis and are considering using kutki, first carefully discuss this with your health-care provider and follow his or her recommendations.

Circulatory/Respiratory	Detoxifier	Digestive	Immune Enhancer	Men's Health
X	X	X		
Metabolic	Nervine	Rejuvenative	Rheumatic	Women's Health

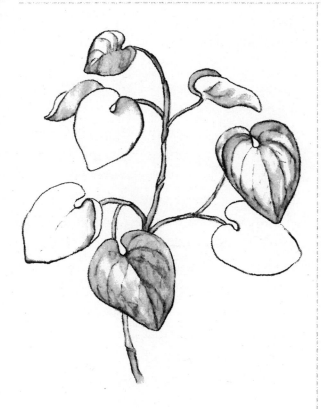

PIPER METHYSTICUM

FAMILIAR: **kava kava, kava**
LATIN: *Piper methysticum*

Kava kava, an ancient medicinal plant indigenous to the South Pacific, has gained recent popularity in the West. Sometimes known as awa by native Hawaiians, extracts of the roots of this tropical plant have been used for ceremonial, recreational, and medicinal purposes by Polynesian natives for millennia. Kava creates a mildly calming euphoric state and appears to avoid the common side effects of many tranquilizing medications.

Kava was traditionally prepared by chewing the root and mixing it with water or coconut milk as part of a ceremonial event. In modern times it is occasionally ingested in ceremonies, but is more commonly consumed as a relaxing beverage and tranquilizing medicine. Modern scientific studies are confirming the beneficial effects of kava in the treatment of anxiety and insomnia, but it should not be used indiscriminately, as rare side effects can occur.

BOTANICAL AND PHYTOCHEMICAL INFORMATION

Kava is a member of the pepper family. A nonclimbing shrub reaching on average up to six feet in height, it has an affinity for warm, swampy areas. Cultivated kava plants no longer produce viable seeds, so the herb is now propagated by way of cuttings throughout the South Pacific and Hawaii. It produces characteristic heart-shaped leaves arising from smooth stems. The underground roots and rhizomes are the source of the medicinal components.

Chemical analyses have determined that both water- and fat-soluble compounds can be extracted from the kava root. The water-soluble components have not been well described, whereas the lipid constituents have been characterized as belonging to a new class of compounds called kava lactones or pyrones. Several of these chemicals, including desmethoxyyangonin, methysticin, and yangonin, have been shown to have pain-relieving and sedating effects through complex actions on the nervous system.

THE SCIENCE OF KAVA

Studies have suggested that almost 50 million Americans struggle with anxiety on a regular basis, and many of today's most widely prescribed drugs are directed toward the treatment of anxiety and insomnia. Unfortunately, most medications for nervousness and sleeping problems carry the side effects of daytime sedation and possible drug dependency. Alternatives to the use of standard anti-anxiety medication would be welcome if they provided relief with fewer adverse

effects. Kava may offer a useful natural option, although it should not be seen as a magic elixir for dissolving the stresses of life. From a holistic perspective, the need for kava should trigger an honest search for the underlying cause of the anxiety or insomnia.

For occasional short-term relief, kava has been shown to be effective in reducing nervousness without the impairment of thinking that usually accompanies tranquilizing drugs. In two studies from Germany, kava was found useful in reducing anxiety without negative reactions after just one week of treatment.[1, 2] In a report of fifty-two outpatients with anxiety, more than 80 percent of those taking kava rated their treatment as "very good" or "good."[3] Another study of forty women going through menopause showed that those taking kava had measurable improvements in their mood and sense of well-being, with significant reductions in both anxiety and depression, when compared with those on a placebo.[4]

Kava may be as effective as many of the standard medications without as many side effects. In a study comparing kava to an anti-anxiety benzodiazepine drug called oxazepam, physiological brain reactions were altered with the medication, but were not affected by kava.[5] Another study looking at the ability of people to identify novel visual stimuli found that subjects given oxazepam performed more poorly than those in a control group, whereas those given kava actually performed better.[6]

Concerns have been raised about kava's potential compounding effects if mixed with alcohol. A German study looking into this issue reported that combining kava with alcohol did not additionally impair performance on a number of neurophysiological tests, and in procedures measuring concentration ability, those subjects taking kava with alcohol actually performed better than those taking alcohol alone.[7] This should not be interpreted as suggesting that you should take kava along with your glass of wine; rather, it highlights the low risk of kava-induced side effects usually associated with sedating substances.

There has been considerable scientific interest into how kava influences the mind and nervous system. Laboratory studies have demonstrated that kava has complex effects on the physiology and chemistry of the brain. Extracts of kava have been shown to dampen the electrical fluctuations of nerve cells.[8] This modulation seems to be through interaction with the receptor for an inhibitory neurochemical known as GABA (gamma-amino-butyric acid).[9] This mechanism is closely related to the way that the common anti-anxiety medications act, but appears to be different enough to avoid many of the common side effects of the standard drugs. Kava's potential therapeutic role in other neurological conditions, ranging from epilepsy to chronic pain to stroke, is just beginning to be explored.[10–12]

THE PRACTICAL USE OF KAVA

Despite its ready availability, kava should be used cautiously, sparingly, and respectfully. For occasional insomnia or an acutely stressful time of life, a short-term course of kava may provide temporary relief. If you are currently taking a prescribed tranquilizer or sleeping medication, discuss the use of kava with your health-care provider before you start it or discontinue your medication. Do not mix kava with any recreational or prescribed drugs that may have sedating effects.

HOW TO USE KAVA

Studies using kava extract have found that doses of 70 to 100 milligrams of kavalactones three times per day are effective in the treatment of mild anxiety. As a sleeping aid, a single dose of 150 to 200 milligrams an hour before bedtime is usually suggested.

One question that has not been fully answered is whether the effectiveness of kava diminishes with repeated use. This issue, known as tolerance, has been investigated in animals and found to be of minor concern. Mice given kava extract daily for weeks showed no tolerance at low dosages and only slight tolerance at high dosages.[13] Despite the minimal loss of efficacy over time, we encourage you not to rely solely on an herbal approach to treat anxiety or insomnia. Do not use kava as a substitute for daily meditation, regular exercise, good nutrition, and healthy emotional choices.

AYURVEDA AND KAVA

From an Ayurvedic perspective, kava can be classified as containing the sweet, bitter, and astringent flavors. It is pacifying to Vata and Pitta, but can be aggravating to Kapha.

PRECAUTIONS

Rare but potentially serious side effects have been reported in people taking kava. Despite its relative safety when taken on its own, it can interact with sedating medications. A report from Georgia described a patient who took kava along with his sedative medication, alprazolam, and became confused and lethargic for several hours.[14] He recovered fully, but did require hospitalization.

A more serious complication of liver injury was reported in a woman taking kava.[15] Her liver tests recovered after the herb was discontinued, and no other cause for her hepatitis could be determined. Another complication, well described among native drinkers of kava, is a skin condition that has been called kava-induced dermopathy.[16] Heavy chronic users of kava can develop thickened, scaly skin. Although it has been suggested that this may represent a niacin deficiency, recent studies have contradicted this explanation.[17] Rare allergic skin reactions have been reported in westerners taking kava extract.[18, 19]

Our bottom line regarding kava is that it is a valuable herbal remedy that may provide an alternative to pharmaceutical anti-anxiety and sleeping medications. However, it should be used appropriately and as part of a holistic program that addresses the underlying issues that contribute to the potential need for kava.

Circulatory/Respiratory	Detoxifier	Digestive	Immune Enhancer	Men's Health
Metabolic	Nervine	Rejuvenative	Rheumatic	Women's Health
	X			

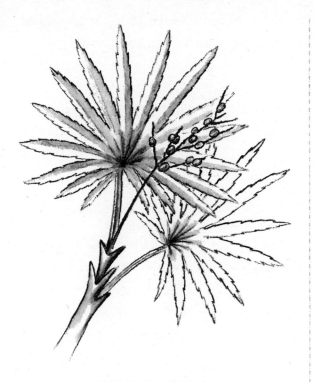

SERENOA
REPENS

FAMILIAR: **saw palmetto**
LATIN: *Serenoa repens, Sabal serrulata,*
Serenoa serrulata

S aw palmetto is a small palm tree native to the southeastern United States. It is found throughout Florida and parts of South Carolina and Mississippi. The berries of this plant were prized by Native Americans as a general tonic, as a treatment for impotence and painful urination in men, and as a natural remedy for infertility and menstrual irregularities in women. Today saw palmetto is one of the most widely used herbal medicines in the treatment of benign prostatic hyperplasia (BPH). This condition, which affects over half of men in their sixties and as many as 90 percent of men in their eighties, accounts for over 350,000 operations each year in the United States. Although saw palmetto is not a cure for this common condition that may cause difficulties with urination, it can improve the quality of life for many men.

BOTANICAL AND PHYTOCHEMICAL INFORMATION

Saw palmetto is a low-growing palm that has sharp, spinelike leaf blades, which account for its common name. The mature plant may reach fifteen to twenty feet in height and may live as long as seven hundred years. Each palm produces clusters of white flowers in the spring that give rise to fruits in the summer. Each plant produces up to five hundred berries that turn from green to orange to deep bluish black over the course of several months.

For years, saw palmetto was viewed as an undesirable plant that was difficult to remove when clearing grazing pastures and farmland. With the growing interest in saw palmetto as a medicinal substance, the economic value of this plant has been recognized. It is now viewed as a cash crop by many of the same landowners that previously saw it as an unwelcome weed.

Tablets and capsules of saw palmetto contain dried berries, often standardized to specific concentrations of sterols or fatty acids. Chemical analyses have identified a variety of free fatty acids in the fruits, including capric, lauric, and oleic acids. Several different medium- and long-chain alcohols and sterols have also been characterized. Although the responsible substances have not yet been identified, it is the fat-soluble components of saw palmetto berries that appear to contain the chemicals that influence the prostate gland.

THE SCIENCE OF SAW PALMETTO

Benign prostatic hyperplasia is a condition in which a man's prostate gland enlarges, at times resulting in the obstruction of the outflow tract from the bladder. The underlying cause of BPH is not fully understood, but seems to be related to the concentration of sex hormones that stimulate the prostate gland. The most important of these hormones is dihydrotestosterone (DHT), which is derived from testosterone. A popular medication for BPH, finasteride, blocks the enzyme that converts testosterone to DHT. Several studies have suggested that one of saw palmetto's actions is to inhibit this same enzyme, possibly accounting in part for its efficacy in the treatment of BPH.[1-3]

The nervous system plays an important role in coordinating normal urinary function, and several drugs used to treat BPH act on the neurological inputs to the lower urinary tact. In addition to its role on hormonal levels, saw palmetto also influences the neurochemicals that coordinate urinary function.[4,5] The effect of these actions is to reduce the spasm that can interfere with normal urination.

Saw palmetto fruits have also demonstrated anti-inflammatory activity. Components of a saw palmetto extract inhibit the formation of inflammatory prostaglandins.[6] This property may also contribute to the value of saw palmetto in the treatment of BPH.

Regardless of how it works, there is convincing evidence that saw palmetto does lead to improvements in urinary function in men with BPH. Saw palmetto seems to help with several aspects of bladder emptying. It can improve urinary flow, decrease discomfort, and reduce the amount of residual urine that is left in the bladder after voiding.[7, 8] A report from Germany found that more than eighty percent of men taking saw palmetto reported a good to excellent response to the herbal extract.[9] A study from Hungary reported that nine out of ten patients on saw palmetto had marked improvements in their ability to empty their bladders.[10] Although not all reports have shown definite objective improvements in urinary function,[11] a recent review of eighteen studies encompassing almost three thousand men found that overall saw palmetto is effective in improving both the symptoms and flow measures of men with BPH.[12] It seems to be as effective as the most popular medication, finasteride, with fewer side effects.

THE PRACTICAL USE OF SAW PALMETTO

In the treatment of BPH, saw palmetto berry extract is usually taken twice daily. Studies have reported an improvement in symptoms in as little as one month after taking the herb, although benefits accrue over the course of three to six months.

In addition to its use in BPH, saw palmetto berries have a traditional rejuvenating role for both men and women. It was used by Native Americans to help people recover from debilitating illnesses or injuries. Saw palmetto was recommended to increase both male and female fertility, although there has not been any scientific evidence to support this property. The berries have a soothing, toning effect on mucous membranes and can be taken for colds and coughs.

HOW TO USE SAW PALMETTO

Saw palmetto extract is now widely available. Most tablets and capsules contain a standardized concentration of fatty acids from 80 to 95 percent. Individual capsules usually contain 80 or 160 milligrams with a daily recommended dose of 320 milligrams. Crude berries are occasionally available, which can be taken at a dose of 10 grams twice daily.

AYURVEDA AND SAW PALMETTO

The fresh berries, which carry the sweet, pungent, and astringent tastes, have a mild warming effect on the physiology. They are pacifying to Vata and Pitta, with the potential to increase Kapha in high doses. The actions of saw palmetto on the urinary system are similar to those of the Ayurvedic herb gokshura (*Tribulis terrestris*).

PRECAUTIONS

Rare digestive distress is associated with saw palmetto ingestion. In contrast to its traditional use for fertility, saw palmetto has been found in laboratory studies to inhibit sperm motility at high concentrations.[13] Although there have not been any reports of clinical fertility problems with saw palmetto, it should probably be avoided by a potential father if pregnancy is desired. Because BPH rarely causes problems before the age of fifty, this potential concern about saw palmetto is usually not relevant.

Circulatory/Respiratory	Detoxifier	Digestive	Immune Enhancer	Men's Health
				X
Metabolic	Nervine	Rejuvenative	Rheumatic	Women's Health

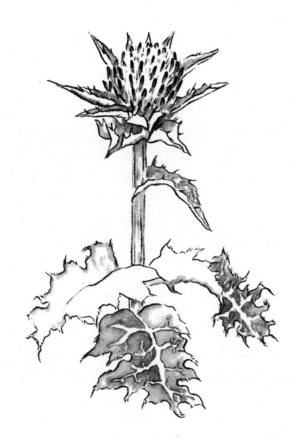

SILYBUM MARIANUM

FAMILIAR: **milk thistle**
LATIN: *Silybum marianum, Carduus marianus*

Milk thistle is an ancient European medicinal herb that has gained modern popularity as a liver protectant. Its name derives from its characteristic white-veined leaves, which, according to legend, contain the milk of the Madonna. Drawing upon the ancient "doctrine of signatures," which holds that nature provides clues to the therapeutic value of a plant, milk thistle was traditionally taken by nursing mothers seeking to improve the quality of their breast milk.

Since the time of the ancient Greeks, milk thistle has been prescribed as a remedy for liver ailments. Physicians throughout medieval times and the Renaissance praised its ability to detoxify the body of "bad bile." As modern researchers began to look seriously at milk thistle, they discovered that it offered genuine value in the treatment of liver disease. It has subsequently become one of the most popular herbs among patients with liver disease.

BOTANICAL AND PHYTOCHEMICAL INFORMATION

Milk thistle is native to the Mediterranean region and grows widely throughout Europe. It was brought to America by early Western European settlers and is now well established in the United States and Latin America. Milk thistle is a member of the Compositae family, which includes chicory, burdock, and artichoke.

The full-grown milk thistle plant can reach five feet in height and is easily recognized by its purple flower heads and spiny, white-veined leaves. The medicinal herb is primarily derived from the small, hard fruits that are often mistakenly referred to as seeds.

The chemical constituent in milk thistle that has been identified as the biologically active substance is called silymarin. Silymarin is composed of several unique flavonoids, the most important of which is silybin. Commercially available milk thistle extracts are usually standardized to contain 70 percent silybin.

Silymarin is easily absorbed from the digestive tract and processed by the liver, where it is concentrated in the bile.[1] This may explain why its potent antioxidant properties seem to have their greatest impact in protecting the liver from toxic and infectious insults.

THE SCIENCE OF MILK THISTLE

Milk thistle has shown promise in a number of medical conditions including diseases of the liver, high cholesterol, and psoriasis. Studies from over thirty years ago on patients with liver damage resulting from a variety of causes found that those taking silymarin were more likely to show both clinical and laboratory improvement than were control subjects.[2,3] Subsequent investigations in people with viral hepatitis have shown that those given milk thistle have faster normalization of liver function tests and more-rapid clinical recoveries.[4] These findings were true for patients with both hepatitis A and hepatitis B infections.

Reports on patients with cirrhosis of the liver who were given silymarin also had encouraging results. People with scarring of their livers due to alcohol or infection who received milk thistle were more likely to live longer than control patients, even though there were not significant changes in laboratory measurements of liver function.[5] Other studies have shown that silymarin also has a beneficial effect in a variety of liver ailments, including injuries from poisonous mushrooms, chemicals, and pharmaceutical drugs.[6,7] Another potentially useful role for silymarin is in the treatment of high cholesterol. Studies in both rats and rabbits have shown that silymarin has a positive effect in normalizing lipid metabolism, reducing serum cholesterol levels and slowing the development of atherosclerosis.[8–10] This effect has yet to be formally studied in people.

THE PRACTICAL USE OF MILK THISTLE

Although milk thistle has many potential therapeutic uses, its predominant modern role is in the treatment of liver disease. The German Commission E has approved it for the treatment of dyspepsia and in the supportive therapy of inflammatory liver conditions and cirrhosis. If you have active or chronic liver disease, discuss the use of milk thistle with your health-care provider. In cases of viral hepatitis, milk thistle may improve both how you feel and the degree of liver function abnormalities as measured by blood tests. If you are recovering from the excessive use of alcohol, a month of silymarin may help your liver to recover more rapidly and completely. If you have been diagnosed with cirrhosis of the liver due to toxic or infectious damage, a trial of milk thistle may be warranted. Although your liver blood tests may not show dramatic improvement, you may feel better.

Theoretically, milk thistle could play a beneficial role in reducing the toxicity to the liver from pharmaceutical drugs, including cancer chemotherapy medicines. Unfortunately, there has not been any formal scientific investigation of milk thistle for this use. Because of its concentration in the liver, you should use silymarin cautiously if you are taking a prescribed medicine that is metabolized by the liver, as it theoretically may alter the level of the drug in your system.

HOW TO USE MILK THISTLE

Milk thistle is widely available in health-food stores, where it is available as tablets and tinctures. Most tablets have between 100 and 300 milligrams of milk thistle standardized to contain 70 percent silymarin. The usual therapeutic dose is between 300 and 800 milligrams of silymarin per day in two or three divided doses. Milk thistle has been used by patients in studies for up to two years continuously without apparent side effects.

AYURVEDA AND MILK THISTLE

The original Ayurvedic sages did not know milk thistle. Although not botanically related, milk thistle, kutki, and phyllanthus have comparable medicinal profiles and are applied in similar clinical conditions. From an Ayurvedic perspective, milk thistle is bitter in taste and carries a cooling potency. It is pacifying to Pitta and Kapha, but can be mildly aggravating to Vata if used for a prolonged time.

PRECAUTIONS

Milk thistle has a remarkable safety profile. Other than the possibility of slightly loose stools, we have not come across any reports of untoward side effects. If you are taking a pharmaceutical agent, discuss the use of milk thistle with your health adviser to monitor any influence it may have on your medication levels.

Circulatory/Respiratory	Detoxifier	Digestive	Immune Enhancer	Men's Health
	X			
Metabolic	Nervine	Rejuvenative	Rheumatic	Women's Health

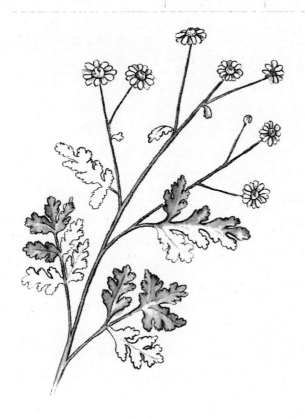

TANACETUM PARTHENIUM

FAMILIAR: **feverfew, bachelor's buttons**
LATIN: *Tanacetum parthenium,*
Chrysanthemum parthenium

Well known to ancient Egyptian and Greek physicians, feverfew received its name for its ability to lower the fever in people facing infections. Sometimes known as "featherfew" in recognition of its feathery leaves, it has a long-standing reputation in the world of natural medicine as an effective pain reliever. Scientific studies over the past thirty years have investigated the traditional claims surrounding feverfew, with most supporting its value, particularly in the prevention of migraine headaches. Other reports have lent credibility to the value of feverfew in the treatment of arthritic conditions.

BOTANICAL AND PHYTOCHEMICAL INFORMATION

Feverfew is related to the chrysanthemum, producing daisylike flowers of white rays on a yellow center. The hardy, perennial feverfew plant grows to about two and one-half feet in height and is widely cultivated in gardens for its attractive leaves and flowers. Native to southern Europe and the Caucasus region between Europe and Asia, it is now found throughout the world in temperate climates. A component of its essential oil has a characteristic pungent odor that repels bees.

The volatile oil of feverfew is chemically complex, containing a variety of organic acids, ethers, and sesquiterpene lactones. The most important constituent appears to be parthenolide, although other natural chemical components play a role in feverfew's therapeutic properties. These chemicals appear to block the production of inflammatory prostaglandins, influence the brain's production of neurochemicals involved in pain regulation, and inhibit blood vessels from going into spasm.

THE SCIENCE OF FEVERFEW

Pharmacological studies since the 1980s have demonstrated that feverfew has potent anti-inflammatory activity, capable of inhibiting the production of prostaglandins.[1–3] Closely associated with its anti-inflammatory effects is feverfew's ability to keep platelets from sticking together and releasing serotonin.[4] Since altered serotonin metabolism has been associated with migraine headaches, this property of feverfew may, in part, explain its efficacy in the treatment of vascular headaches. Other chemicals contained in feverfew, including melatonin, may also play a role.[5]

Regardless of what components may be pharmacologically active, the real question concerns feverfew's effectiveness in the treatment of migraine headaches. A recent review of published studies found that three of five reports showed significant benefits of feverfew over a placebo, with one of the two negative studies providing only minimal data to substantiate its conclusion.[6] In the majority of reports, the frequency of migraines and the severity of headache pain diminished in the patients taking feverfew.[7–9] In addition to reducing the headache, feverfew helped diminish the associated symptoms of nausea and light and noise sensitivity. In one study comparing people taking feverfew with those on a placebo, the mean number of monthly headaches decreased from more than seven to less than two.[10] In another study of seventy-six patients, there was, on average, about a 25-percent reduction in the number of headache attacks in those taking the equivalent of two medium-sized feverfew leaves per day.[11] Side effects were generally mild, consisting of mouth sores, mild digestive symptoms, and an occasional rebound increase in headaches when feverfew was discontinued.

Feverfew is considered useful as a preventative migraine medicine rather than as a treatment once the headache has established itself. The benefits of feverfew may be seen as early as during the first months of treatment. It is important to realize that for most people feverfew does not completely eliminate migraines; rather, it reduces their frequency and severity.

The role of feverfew in other health conditions has not been well studied. One of its traditional uses has been in the treatment of inflammatory arthritic conditions, but the one modern study that researched its role in rheumatoid arthritis failed to demonstrate any definite value.[12]

One concern regarding studies on feverfew is the variable content of active ingredients in different batches of the herb. Researchers from England, looking at many different formulations of feverfew, found levels of parthenolide ranging from none to almost 1 percent of the herbal dose.[13] Whether the lack of active constituent is due to misidentification of the herb, deterioration over time, or intentional substitution, these findings emphasize the need for quality control and standardization in the herbal industry. Most feverfew formulations available in the United States are now standardized to contain between .2 percent and .9 percent parthenolides.

THE PRACTICAL USE OF FEVERFEW

Migraines are characterized by throbbing pain, often associated with nausea and sensitivity to loud sounds and bright lights. Anyone with more than an occasional headache should have a thorough medical evaluation to rule out other conditions that may cause headaches. Although there are many effective medications available for the prevention and symptomatic treatment of migraines, many people prefer to take a holistic approach.

If you are susceptible to frequent migraine headaches, feverfew may be worth a trial. You will likely need to take it daily for at least a month before noticing a reduction in the frequency or intensity of your headaches. It will not have much value if you take it during a migraine attack. Before beginning any medicine or herbal remedy for migraines, first evaluate the basic aspects of your lifestyle. Be sure you are getting enough rest, and that you are eating well and have eliminated alcohol and caffeine from your diet. Look at the chronic and acute stresses in your life, and take steps to reduce them. Although there are genetic components to migraine susceptibility, lifestyle issues can have a major impact.

HOW TO USE FEVERFEW

Feverfew is easy to grow in your garden, and a few leaves can be taken daily to prevent headaches. Tablets and capsules of the herb are widely available, but make certain that you are obtaining feverfew from a reputable source that offers a standardized formulation. Clinical studies have used a daily dose of dried feverfew leaves in the range of 50 to 100 milligrams. Depending upon the concentration of the preparation, this is equivalent to about 2 milligrams of parthenolide. Most commercially available capsules contain between 80 and 250 milligrams of dried feverfew, with a recommended dose of between two and four capsules per day.

If you are growing your own, two to three fresh feverfew leaves daily are usually sufficient to produce a therapeutic benefit. The flowering tops contain the highest concentration of parthenolide, closely followed by the leaves. The stems and roots have only minimal amounts of the presumed active constituent.

AYURVEDA AND FEVERFEW

Feverfew was not an original Ayurvedic herb, but can be understood according to Ayurvedic principles. It has a predominantly bitter taste and a cooling influence on the system. It is helpful in reducing Pitta and Kapha, but may be aggravating to Vata. According to Ayurveda, migraine headaches are usually a Pitta aggravation, as opposed to tension headaches, which are usually more Vata. In our personal experience, we have seen both Pitta and Vata imbalances respond to feverfew.

PRECAUTIONS

Some people are sensitive to chemical components of feverfew. A small percentage of regular users who chew feverfew leaves will develop mouth sores, although, in one study, people taking the placebo actually reported this problem more often than those taking feverfew. People tending gardens with feverfew occasionally develop an allergic skin reaction.

Although we have not seen any modern reports, one of feverfew's traditional uses was to induce menstruation, so pregnant women should avoid it. Because of its ability to inhibit platelet aggregation in laboratory studies, people taking blood-thinning medications should not take feverfew.

Circulatory/Respiratory	Detoxifier	Digestive	Immune Enhancer	Men's Health
Metabolic	Nervine	Rejuvenative	Rheumatic	Women's Health
	X		X ?	

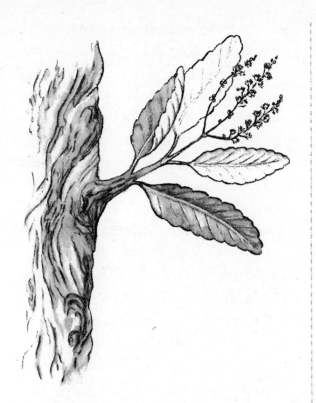

TERMINALIA
ARJUNA

FAMILIAR: **arjuna myrobalan**
LATIN: *Terminalia arjuna*
SANSKRIT: arjuna

The arjuna tree, which grows throughout India, has been valued for its therapeutic properties since the original Ayurvedic writings thousands of years ago. It is revered both for its wood and as a source of herbal medicine. The myth surrounding arjuna relates that the two sons of the Tree Spirit King insulted a wizard, who turned them both into arjuna trees. Even in modern times, in recognition of their enchanted heritage, lumbermen perform rituals of respect before cutting arjuna trees.[1]

Arjuna's traditional use has been as a heart tonic, with modern studies supporting its therapeutic role in cardiac conditions. It has effects on the circulatory system ranging from the lowering of cholesterol levels to improving the strength of heart contractions.

BOTANICAL AND PHYTOCHEMICAL INFORMATION

Arjuna is a beautiful deciduous tree that can reach heights of one hundred feet. It grows throughout the sub-Himalayan region of India and Sri Lanka, preferring wet, marshy regions. The arjuna tree has ovoid leaves and produces clusters of small white flowers. It is the inner layers of its silver-white bark that are used for medicinal purposes.

Arjuna's bark contains amino acids, phenols, nitrates, and tannins. Ellagic acid, a chemical constituent of arjuna, has been shown to protect DNA strands from mutations. Arjunin, a unique tannin isolated from arjuna, may also have potential anticancer properties. The chemical components responsible for arjuna's effects on the circulatory system have not yet been identified.

THE SCIENCE OF ARJUNA

Arjuna is good example of an herb whose traditional use inspired scientific research that confirmed its historical value. Studies around the world have demonstrated beneficial effects of arjuna on important aspects of the cardiovascular system. Animal studies have shown that arjuna can substantially lower serum cholesterol levels and improve the HDL:cholesterol ratio without significant side effects.[2, 3]

People with known coronary artery disease who took arjuna showed a significant reduction in the number of anginal chest pain episodes along with a reduction in their blood pressure.[4] Arjuna was not effective in heart patients with unstable angina pectoris, but was able to reduce by half the anginal episodes in patients with stable heart disease. In patients with a history of heart attacks and impairment in heart muscle function, arjuna was associated with a reduction in the frequency of chest pain attacks and improvement in the ability of their heart muscles to contract.[5] Another study of people with congestive heart failure found that those taking arjuna improved in several measures of cardiac function.[6] They also showed sustained enhancement in their overall functioning and quality of life. When combined with guggulu, arjuna was shown to protect the heart muscle in animals when subjected to cardiac-damaging drugs.[7]

Although the benefits of arjuna appear to be substantial, its appropriate role in the modern treatment of heart disease remains to be defined. Cardiovascular disease is a serious health concern, representing the number-one cause of death in Western society. An herbal approach that may improve the quality of life for people with heart disease is worthy of serious consideration by the medical community. On the other hand, if you have heart disease, it is not the time to experiment on your own with an herbal medicine that may interact with the pharmaceutical drugs you are taking. Our recommendation, if you have coronary artery disease, is that you use an herbal approach only under the close supervision of your physician. You may wish to refer your doctor to the articles referenced in this book for his or her consideration.

In addition to its role in heart disease, arjuna has shown other potentially beneficial effects. It can inhibit the growth of certain cancer cell lines and has antibiotic activity against several disease-causing germs, including the bacteria that cause gonorrhea.[8, 9] Traditionally, arjuna has been used to regulate blood sugar, treat skin sores, and help heal bone fractures. These properties have yet to be scientifically investigated.

THE PRACTICAL USE OF ARJUNA

In Ayurvedic medicine, the astringent properties of arjuna are applied to conditions that require the clearing of toxins and the healing of wounds. In addition to its use in heart disease, arjuna is often prescribed for disorders of the digestive tract, including acute gallbladder and liver diseases, diarrhea, and dysentery. In such cases a strong tea is given three times daily until the symptoms improve.

It is a useful topical herb for skin conditions including wounds and ulcers. In the case of acne, a paste applied directly to a sore and left to dry can help clear the infection and stimulate healing. Arjuna is traditionally used to treat people who bruise easily, although whether it works on blood vessels or the clotting system has not been researched. Its cleansing and hemostatic properties are also applied to people with bleeding gums, who are encouraged to gargle with a suspension of powdered bark.

HOW TO USE ARJUNA

Arjuna is not yet readily available in the West, although an increasing number of Ayurvedic heart tonics contain arjuna as their first ingredient. It is available in bulk powdered form from herbal importers.

The standard dose for heart disease is 500 milligrams three times daily. Tradi-

tionally it is mixed with warm milk and sugar. For digestive disorders, arjuna is prepared as a tea with one teaspoon per cup of hot water taken every six hours until the diarrhea or cramping has passed.

As a topical wash for sores, a decoction can be prepared by boiling one tablespoon of arjuna powdered bark in two cups of water until the volume is reduced in half. Wash the wound with the liquid several times a day. This same formula can be used as a mouthwash or gargle. As a treatment for acne, arjuna powder is mixed with water to make a paste that can be directly applied to the skin lesion.

AYURVEDA AND ARJUNA

The predominant taste of arjuna is astringent, with a slightly pungent secondary component. It has a cooling, anti-inflammatory influence on the physiology. It is pacifying to both Pitta and Kapha, but may increase Vata after prolonged usage.

PRECAUTIONS

Serious side effects have not been reported with arjuna. If you are considering arjuna in the hope that it may help with your heart disease, it is absolutely essential that you first discuss it with your heart doctor. You should not stop any heart medication before starting arjuna, and you should be closely monitored by your health-care provider.

Circulatory/Respiratory	Detoxifier	Digestive	Immune Enhancer	Men's Health
X	X	X		
Metabolic	Nervine	Rejuvenative	Rheumatic	Women's Health

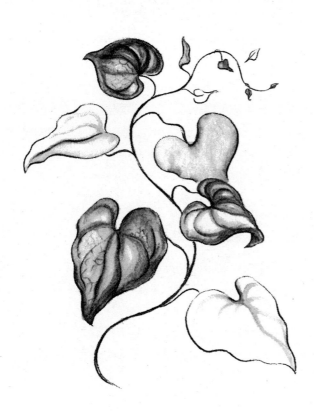

TINOSPORA CORDIFOLIA

FAMILIAR: **amrit, heart-leaved moonseed**

LATIN: *Tinospora cordifolia*

SANSKRIT: amrit, guduchi

A classical Vedic myth relates that the ancient gods churned the primordial ocean, producing an ambrosial nectar that conferred immortality on any being that partook of it. This nectar was called *amrit,* meaning "imperishable." The application of this powerful name to this native Indian plant reflects its position in the Ayurvedic pharmacy as a valued tonic herb, conferring vitality and the energy of youth. Although modern studies cannot yet confirm its immortalizing qualities, there is an expanding body of research to suggest that amrit does offer broad health-promoting properties.

BOTANICAL AND PHYTOCHEMICAL INFORMATION

Tinospora cordifolia is an attractive perennial creeping plant with heart-shaped leaves. It favors shady, damp environments and tends to grow among hedge bushes. Amrit has a papery, light gray bark and small yellow flowers. The leaves, stems, and roots are all used medicinally.

Several characteristic bitter principles have been identified in amrit. Various glycosides and terpenes, including unique compounds called tinosporine and cordifolisides A, B, and C, have been isolated from alcohol and water extracts of its stems and leaves.

THE SCIENCE OF AMRIT

Many studies have evaluated the effects of amrit on the immune system. Laboratory studies have shown that amrit can enhance the production of antibodies and improve the function of macrophages, the cells responsible for gobbling up foreign proteins.[1] In animals that receive immune-toxic drugs, amrit helps restore the production of natural immune-enhancing chemicals such as interferon and tumor necrosis factor (TNF).[2] Animals with serious infections given amrit are able to more effectively clear the bacteria, resulting in more rapid and complete recovery. *Tinospora cordifolia* does not appear to have direct antibiotic activity; rather, it seems to stimulate the host's immune defense system to function more effectively.[3] This has been shown to be true against fungal and parasitic as well as bacterial infections.[4, 5]

The immune-potentiating properties of amrit have been applied to people undergoing surgery. A series of reports from Bombay, India, have shown that patients receiving an amrit extract prior to major abdominal surgery had fewer postoperative infections and significantly improved outcomes, compared against those receiving standard surgical care.[6, 7] Studies to determine why those patients did so much better found that the white blood cells of those who received amrit were better able to engulf and eliminate disease-causing bacteria.[8]

Amrit has also demonstrated potentially useful properties in cancer. A recent study reported that amrit killed tumor cells very effectively when added to a culture of cancer cells.[9] In another animal study, amrit was shown to have potent antioxidant properties that substantially reduced the side effects of a cancer chemotherapy drug on the blood-producing cells in bone marrow.[10] These different properties paint an interesting picture of amrit's potential therapeutic effects. It strengthens natural immunity, may have anticancer activity, and is capable of protecting healthy cells from toxic influences. Reports have also suggested that amrit helps to stabilize blood sugar and lower cholesterol levels.[11, 12]

Amrit can be classified as an adaptogen, a substance that helps the individual adapt more readily to life challenges. This class of herbs, which includes ginseng and ashwagandha, offers protection against the deleterious health effects from a wide range of stresses. An example of its protective properties is a recent study that showed amrit was able to reduce the harmful action of the chemotherapy drug cisplatin on the digestive tract.[13] It limited the extent of damage to the stomach lining, normalized gastric emptying, and stabilized intestinal function. With no reported serious side effects, amrit is a prime candidate for further scientific research as an agent that can enhance the body's recuperative powers.

THE PRACTICAL USE OF AMRIT

Amrit is just beginning to become available in the West. It is usually a component of Ayurvedic formulas designed to enhance immunity and modify a person's response to stress. Its traditional role has been in the treatment of infectious illnesses, ranging from colds to syphilis. It is rejuvenative as well as detoxifying. Amrit is often a component of formulas used in the treatment of chronic skin disorders such as psoriasis or eczema, although we have not seen any scientific studies that have quantified its role in dermatological conditions. It is also reported to be one of the best herbal medicines for gout.

HOW TO USE AMRIT

Tinospora cordifolia is available in powdered form from herbal importers. The usual dosage for immune enhancement is one teaspoon twice daily. This can be taken on a maintenance basis if you are facing a persistent challenge such as cancer, or can be used at the onset of a cold or flu to be taken for a week. It can be combined with shatavari or ashwagandha as a general tonic, or with aloe vera juice as part of a detoxifying formula. It can also be made into a paste and applied directly to chronic skin irritations.

AYURVEDA AND AMRIT

Amrit contains the bitter, pungent, and astringent tastes. It has a heating potency with a sweet post-digestive effect. It is classically used to clear the system of excessive Pitta accumulation, but is balancing to all three doshas.

PRECAUTIONS

No significant adverse effects have been reported with amrit. It can be slightly constipating if used for a prolonged time by people who are prone to sluggish bowels.

Circulatory/Respiratory	Detoxifier	Digestive	Immune Enhancer	Men's Health
	X		X	
Metabolic	Nervine	Rejuvenative	Rheumatic	Women's Health
		X		

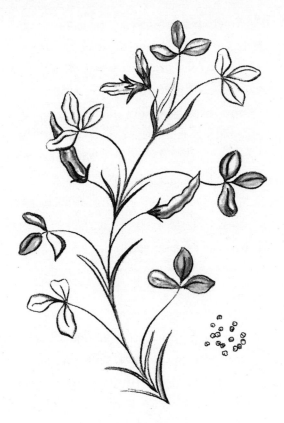

TRIGONELLA FOENUM-GRAECUM

FAMILIAR: **fenugreek**
LATIN: *Trigonella foenum-graecum*
SANSKRIT/HINDI: methi

Fenugreek is one of the earliest spices used by human beings for culinary and medicinal purposes. Native to the lands that surround the Arabian Sea, fenugreek was known to the ancient Egyptian and Greek physicians, and was valued by Hippocrates in the fifth century B.C. A member of the legume family, fenugreek is now cultivated in the Middle East, India, China, and Greece. With its distinctive aroma, fenugreek is commonly added to perfumes, candies, and curried spice blends. It has traditional therapeutic value as a nutritive tonic and in the treatment of digestive disorders and respiratory complaints. Scientific studies have shown fenugreek to be beneficial in lowering elevated blood sugar and cholesterol levels.

BOTANICAL AND PHYTOCHEMICAL INFORMATION

Fenugreek is an annual herb that grows to about two feet in height. The Latin name *Trigonella,* meaning "three-angled," refers to the oval-shaped leaves that grow in triad clusters. The plant produces white flowers in the early summer that give rise to sickle-shaped pods, containing ten to twenty yellow seeds. The leaves and pods are used medicinally.

Chemical analysis of the seeds reveals a strong-smelling volatile oil, a mucilaginous polysaccharide, and a variety of alkaloids and flavonoids. Several unique saponins called trigoneosides have been identified. Diosgenin, a saponin also present in wild yams, is synthesized into female hormones used in birth-control pills and hormone-replacement therapy. Over 25 percent of the seed is composed of fiber. It has been suggested that the fiber and saponins are responsible for fenugreek's cholesterol-lowering action, by binding cholesterol in the digestive tract so it cannot be fully absorbed into the bloodstream.[1]

THE SCIENCE OF FENUGREEK

Fenugreek has been most researched for its effect on blood glucose levels. Many studies in diabetic animals have shown that the leaves and ground seeds of fenugreek lower blood sugar levels.[2-4] The ability of fenugreek to lower glucose levels may be due to its content of an amino acid (4-hydroxyisoleucine) that stimulates the release of insulin.[5]

The effects of fenugreek on blood sugar levels have been shown to be relevant to human beings. Insulin-dependent diabetics given fenugreek seed powder with breakfast and dinner showed reduced fasting blood sugar levels and improved glucose tolerance tests.[6] They also had a lowering of their cholesterol and triglyceride levels. In another study, patients with mild noninsulin-dependent diabetes given fenugreek at a dose of 2.5 grams twice daily showed a significant reduction in their blood sugar levels.[7] Other patients with coronary artery disease given fenugreek for three months showed lower cholesterol and triglyceride levels. In this report from India, healthy people without diabetes or heart disease given fenugreek did not demonstrate any change in their sugar or cholesterol values.

Fenugreek's effect on cholesterol was predicted by an earlier animal study that found an extract able to reduce blood cholesterol levels by about 25 percent in rats over a one-month period.[8] This cholesterol-lowering effect is in part due to the binding of cholesterol by the fiber component of the seeds. The saponins present in fenugreek may also play a role by blocking the absorption of bile acids that carry cholesterol into the bloodstream.

An interesting feature of fenugreek is its ability to increase appetite, resulting in greater food conusmption.[9] Although this may not sound appealing for people trying to lose weight, it can be a valuable aid for people with chronic illness or depression who have trouble consuming enough daily calories to support their recovery. It is interesting that despite its appetite-enhancing effects, fenugreek is able to lower serum cholesterol levels.

In addition to its glucose- and cholesterol-lowering effects, fenugreek leaves have demonstrated antioxidant and pain-relieving effects.[10,11] Although the leaves are not well known in the West, they are used in a manner similar to spinach in the Middle East and India. The antioxidant properties may be due to their rich content of vitamin C and beta-carotene.[12] Another traditional use for fenugreek leaves and seeds in Saudi Arabia is in the treatment of kidney stones. A study in animals found that rats receiving fenugreek daily for a month had a significant reduction in the quantity of calcium oxalate deposited in their kidneys, supporting its folk medicine use.[13] It's obvious that this pungent spice has many potential health-promoting benefits, worthy of further scientific investigation.

THE PRACTICAL USE OF FENUGREEK

Fenugreek is best consumed as part of a balanced diet. If you have elevated cholesterol levels or suffer with diabetes, try to get a couple of teaspoons of fenugreek into your diet on a daily basis. A teaspoonful in a cup of hot milk, sweetened with honey, before bedtime can help induce sound sleep. Fenugreek tea taken after a meal can be soothing to an upset stomach. One of the herb's traditional uses has been to increase the quantity of breast milk in nursing mothers. Other than making mom smell a little like maple syrup, it seems to be well tolerated and moderately effective.

HOW TO USE FENUGREEK

Fenugreek seeds are usually available at grocery stores, although you may need to go to a Middle Eastern or Indian spice shop to find it as an individual spice, rather than as part of a curry blend.

Health-food stores usually carry ground seeds in capsule form with about 500 milligrams per dose. To make a digestion-settling tea, simmer two teaspoons of crushed or ground seeds in a cup of hot water. As a gargle for sore throats and colds, boil two teaspoons in a cup of water down to one-half cup and use while still warm.

As an aid to lowering cholesterol, take one gram twice daily, either as a powder mixed in food or liquid, or in the form of tablets. Anecdotal reports of fenugreek to increase breast milk suggest that 2 to 8 grams in divided doses can enhance lactation. Be sure to drink plenty of water if you are using fenugreek for this purpose.

The ground seeds can be made into a paste with water and used as a poultice in the treatment of skin eruptions. A fenugreek paste is used to draw out infection from boils and can be applied directly to acne lesions, left until dry, and then washed off.

AYURVEDA AND FENUGREEK

The bitter taste predominates in fenugreek, followed by pungent and sweet. The net effect of fenugreek on the physiology is heating. It is pacifying to Vata and Kapha, but has the potential of aggravating Pitta if taken in excess.

PRECAUTIONS

Fenugreek should generally be avoided during pregnancy, as it may have a stimu-lating effect on the uterus. Rare allergic reactions have been described, but considering its long-standing worldwide use, it is a very safe culinary and medicinal spice.[14]

Circulatory/Respiratory	Detoxifier	Digestive	Immune Enhancer	Men's Health
		X		
Metabolic	Nervine	Rejuvenative	Rheumatic	Women's Health
X		X		

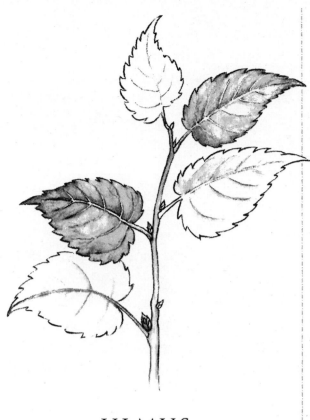

ULMUS
RUBRA

FAMILIAR: **slippery elm**
LATIN: *Ulmus rubra*

Slippery elm is a wonderful medicinal herb that is an American original. Prized by Native Americans, it was embraced by early settlers for its value as both a food source and medicine. Although introduced to Europe in the seventeenth century, it never received wide acceptance. In America, however, slippery elm was included for over a century in our official pharmacopoeia, and remains on the FDA's "safe and effective" list. Nevertheless, there are no formal scientific studies published on it.

Traditionally, slippery elm has been used for a wide range of health concerns, whenever there is evidence of inflammation. Its soothing mucilaginous qualities have been applied to conditions ranging from sore throat to inflamed hemorrhoids. A popular ingredient in modern herbal teas and throat lozenges, slippery elm is one of nature's gentlest healing allies.

BOTANICAL AND PHYTOCHEMICAL INFORMATION

The slippery elm tree is native to North America, where both the outer and inner bark are harvested. Its Latin name *Ulmus rubra,* meaning "red elm," refers to the reddish color of its inner bark. It grows best in soil that has been disturbed, such as abandoned farmland. Slippery elm is susceptible to Dutch elm disease, a fungal infection spread by bark beetles, but less so than other species of elm.

It is primarily the inner bark that is used medicinally. It contains many different sugars, terpenes, and sterols that result in its mucilaginous properties. A fine powder of the bark can be taken internally as a nutritious gruel, made into throat lozenges, or applied as a poultice to irritated skin. Slippery elm's natural mucilage binds to and protects internally and externally inflamed membranes.

THE SCIENCE OF SLIPPERY ELM

Slippery elm is used industrially in many food and medicinal products. It serves as binder material in suppositories, as a demulcent in throat lozenges, and as a thickener in creams and ointments. Slippery elm also serves as an antioxidant preservative in cooking oils. With the many benefits attributed to this herb, it is surprising that it has been ignored by modern medical science. Perhaps it has been overlooked because it is on the boundary between food and natural medicine.

PRACTICAL USES FOR SLIPPERY ELM

Slippery elm has many diverse uses. Native Americans found it beneficial in the treatment of cough and sore throat. Its lubricating qualities loosen and mobilize secretions throughout the respiratory tract. It also has therapeutic effects on the digestive system, where it acts as a gentle bowel tonic, useful in the treatment of both diarrhea and constipation. Heartburn and peptic ulcers respond to the soothing influence of slippery elm, which can cool inflamed mucous membranes. It has properties very similar to marshmallow, which is widely used in Europe for inflammatory problems.

Native American women taught early European settlers the value of slippery elm in easing the pain of childbirth. In addition to its internal use, slippery elm was externally applied to lubricate the birth passage. It was also used after delivery to soothe swollen and irritated vaginal tissues.

Mixed with brown sugar or maple syrup, slippery elm makes a gruel of the kind that sustained early American explorers. George Washington and his armies used it as a source of nutrition during the revolutionary war. It can be helpful in people who are convalescing from an illness and is even digestible by babies.

Slippery elm's benefits extend beyond the digestive system. It is useful in cooling inflamed membranes of the urinary tract. Chronic bladder inflammation, prostatitis, and urethritis have traditionally responded to slippery elm. Its anti-inflammatory qualities can also be recommended for rheumatic conditions, including degenerative arthritis and gout.

Externally, slippery elm can be applied to sores, wounds, and burns. It can be used to treat cold sores, eczema, and festering insect bites. A dilute solution of a slippery elm infusion may help soothe inflamed eyes. A poultice made with powdered slippery elm bark can be applied directly to painful, swollen hemorrhoids, which may also benefit from the internal use of this lubricating substance.

In patients receiving treatment for cancer, we recommend slippery elm to reduce the discomfort of inflamed mucous membranes, a common side effect of chemotherapy or radiation. Made into a porridge with milk, cinnamon, and honey, slippery elm can also provide a nourishing nutritional supplement.

Externally, slippery elm can be combined with comfrey and applied directly to slow-healing skin ulcers. Mixed with cocoa butter or olive oil, it is a soothing sunburn remedy.

HOW TO USE SLIPPERY ELM

As a tea, one ounce of slippery elm bark is added to one pint of hot water and steeped for five minutes. To use the powdered inner bark as a nutritive gruel, boil one tablespoon in a cup of milk and season with brown sugar and cinnamon. As an external poultice, soak the shredded bark in equal parts of hot water and apply directly to the site of irritation. Slippery elm throat lozenges are widely available at most health-food stores; these can be used for relief of a sore throat or prior to a public speaking or singing event.

An ointment can be made by combining one ounce of slippery elm bark powder with three ounces of cocoa or jojoba butter and massaging into the inflamed area. To make a paste, mix powdered bark with purified water until it is the consistency of thick oatmeal, and apply to the irritated skin. Leave it on until it has fully dried, then rinse it off with room-temperature water. This can be repeated three to four times per day until the burn or sore has healed.

AYURVEDA AND SLIPPERY ELM

Although not described in the classic Ayurvedic texts, slippery elm can be classified as possessing sweet and cooling properties, effective in the treatment of excessive Pitta and Vata. Although it can increase Kapha in high doses, it has a mucus-mobilizing effect that can benefit people with asthma, chronic bronchitis, and upper respiratory infections. Highly nutritive, it is used in states of tissue depletion. Slippery elm can restore balance to the blood and heal the mucous membranes of the lungs and stomach.

PRECAUTIONS

The gruel can be slightly difficult to digest in large amounts. At usual doses, slippery elm is a safe, gentle herbal aid.

Circulatory/Respiratory	Detoxifier	Digestive	Immune Enhancer	Men's Health
X		X		
Metabolic	Nervine	Rejuvenative	Rheumatic	Women's Health
		X		

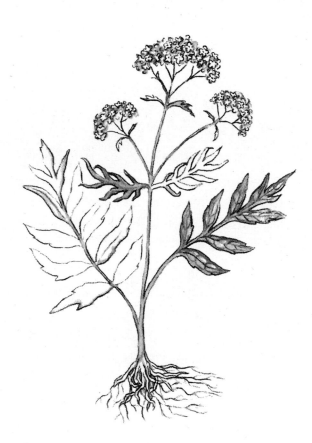

VALERIANA OFFICINALIS

FAMILIAR: **valerian**
LATIN: *Valeriana officinalis, Valeriana jatamansi, Nardostachys jatamansi*
SANSKRIT: tagara, jatamansi

Effective for quieting an overactive mind, valerian has played the role of a natural sedative for millennia. Valerian species have been valued for their calming influence by healers in Asia, Europe, and North America. Dozens of modern studies have confirmed that this strong-smelling herb has measurable tranquilizing properties with minimal side effects.

Widely available in tablets, teas, and tinctures, valerian is approved by the German Commission E as a safe sleep-inducing substance and by the United States Food and Drug Administration as a food and beverage flavoring. Although modern studies have focused primarily on its sleep-inducing effects, valerian also has potential value in the treatment of muscle spasms and hypertension.

BOTANICAL AND PHYTOCHEMICAL INFORMATION

Valerian is a perennial shrub that grows to a height of about four feet. It has clusters of small pink flowers that blossom on long stems. The roots and rhizome are the primary source for the herbal medicine. They contain the unique chemicals known as valeprotriates and valeric acid that appear to be responsible for valerian's calming properties.

Both water- and alcohol-extracted components of valerian root have sedative activity. Even aromatherapy with valerian essential oil can have a calming effect. One of the possible mechanisms for valerian's tranquilizing effect is its ability to increase levels of an inhibitory brain chemical called gamma amino-butyric acid or GABA. Benzodiazepine drugs, such as Valium and Ativan, act on receptors for GABA in the brain, suggesting that the action of valerian may be similar.[1] Other important neurochemicals, including dopamine and serotonin, are also influenced by valerian, so its effects on the brain may be more complex than was initially believed.

THE SCIENCE OF VALERIAN

Valerian has an established history of safety and efficacy. It is one of the most popular herbs in Europe, with over 100 million units prescribed in Germany between 1974 and 1993.[2] Studies from around the world have demonstrated that valerian taken before bedtime can improve the quality of rest a person receives. A report from Sweden demonstrated that valerian was substantially more effective than a placebo in enhancing sleep without side effects.[3] Brain-wave studies of people receiving valerian have shown that it increases the amount of time people spend in the deeper stages of sleep.[4] Other studies have shown that valerian reduces the time it takes to fall asleep, reduces the number of times a person awakens during the night, improves the quality of rest gained during the night, and produces minimal or no drowsiness in the morning.[5, 6]

Animal studies have confirmed that valerian has measurable calming effects. Valerian can prolong the effects of sedative medication and reduce the withdrawal symptoms of animals given tranquilizers for one month.[7, 8] Supporting the relevance of these findings to people, a pharmacist from New Zealand recently reported success in using herbal medicines, including valerian, in a drug detoxification unit.[9]

Studies have suggested that valerian may have stress-neutralizing effects that extend beyond its capacity to promote sound sleep. There are reports that it may diminish the risk of stress ulcers and reduce spasms in the digestive tract.[10, 11] Valerian may also have lipid-lowering effects, with one study demonstrating that extracts of Indian valerian lower total cholesterol levels and raise the HDL (good) component.[12] Finally, extracts of valerian have also been shown to have antibiotic activity against a variety of molds.[13]

PRACTICAL USES FOR VALERIAN

Valerian is useful as a natural relaxant. Although it has not been shown to have any serious long-term side effects, we do not encourage the chronic use of valerian for the treatment of insomnia or anxiety. If you are consistently having trouble sleeping, look to the underlying cause. Are you stressed at work? Are there relationship issues that need to be addressed? Valerian is a valuable botanical gift, but should not be thought of as a substitute for tranquilizing drugs, taken chronically to cope with unresolved emotional imbalances in your life.

Valerian can be helpful in the occasional treatment of sleep difficulties, muscle tension, and mild functional digestive imbalances. As a natural bridge across stressful life challenges, it is a gentle stress-relieving ally.

Valerian has traditionally been used in the treatment of health conditions related to stress, such as heart palpitations, mildly elevated blood pressure, and tension headaches. Although there have not been scientific studies to confirm these benefits of valerian, it is worth a short trial of the herb if you are experiencing intermittent stress-related symptoms. Be certain to discuss your use of valerian with your health-care provider. If valerian is effective in reducing your physical symptoms, it is a good sign that taking other stress-reducing measures, such as meditation, regular exercise, or massage, may be more effective in the long run.

HOW TO USE VALERIAN

Valerian is widely available in tablets and capsules at health-food stores. Studies have suggested that a 450-milligram dose is as effective as 900 milligrams in people taking valerian to help induce sleep.[14] A cup of valerian tea at bedtime, sweetened with honey, can also be helpful. In India, valerian root is used as a potpourri pillow. Children or adults inhale the distinctive fragrance of valerian at bedtime to induce sound sleep.

For anxiety or other stress-related conditions, valerian can be taken three times a day, not to exceed a daily dose of two grams. If you are using valerian more than a few days in a row, ask what more you can do to address the underlying tension in your life.

AYURVEDA AND VALERIAN

Ayurveda recognizes two different medicinal plants in the valerian family: tagara and jatamansi. Tagara is closest to *Valeriana officinalis,* which is the plant most widely used in Western herbal formulas. Jatamansi sometimes goes by the Latin name *Valeriana jatamansi* and is also called *Nardostachys jatamansi.* It is said to be slightly less sedating than tagara, but this has not been confirmed scientifically.

Both are bitter, sweet, pungent, and astringent, although tagara is warming in potency whereas jatamansi is somewhat cooling. Tagara is better for Vata and Kapha, while jatamansi has particular value in pacifying the overheated ruminating mind that excessive Pitta can generate.

PRECAUTIONS

There has been one reported case of a person taking twenty times the recommended dose of valerian and showing mild symptoms of oversedation that fully resolved within a day.[15] Although there have been concerns about morning drowsiness after taking valerian, a recent study comparing valerian with a standard sleeping medicine, flunitrazepam, found a hangover effect from the drug, but not from valerian.[16] There was a very mild decrease in alertness within a couple hours after taking valerian.

Although these effects are subtle, we do not recommend driving a car or operating machinery if you are taking valerian during the day. Also, do not use valerian without the approval of your health-care provider if you are taking any prescribed sedative or tranquilizing medication.

Circulatory/Respiratory	Detoxifier	Digestive	Immune Enhancer	Men's Health
Metabolic	Nervine	Rejuvenative	Rheumatic	Women's Health
	X			

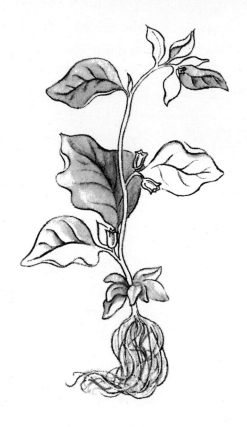

WITHANIA
SOMNIFERA

FAMILIAR: **winter cherry**
LATIN: *Withania somnifera*
SANSKRIT: ashwagandha

Ashwagandha is among the most important herbs in the Ayurvedic pharmacy. Classically known for its rejuvenative benefits, it is the subject of considerable modern scientific attention. It has recently been referred to as "Indian ginseng" for its reputed restorative benefits, although these two timeless tonics, ginseng and ashwagandha, are botanically unrelated.

In Sanskrit, the name *ashwagandha* means "the smell of a horse," implying that this aromatic herb provides the strength of a stallion. It has a traditional use in supporting rejuvenation after illness and as a sexual enhancer for both men and women. Ashwagandha is sometimes referred to as an aphrodisiac, which in Ayurveda is a term applied to substances that enhance the quality of reproductive tissues as well as enlivening sexual potency. Ashwagandha is the primary rasayana, or rejuvenative, for masculine energy.

BOTANICAL AND PHYTOCHEMICAL INFORMATION

Although the leaves and fruit of ashwagandha have therapeutic value, most of the herbal medicine available in the West is derived from the roots of the shrub. The plant, native to India, northern Africa, and the Middle East, is now cultivated in temperate climates around the world, including the United States.

Ashwagandha contains many chemical constituents, including unique compounds called withanolides. The medicinal components have been characterized as steroidal alkaloids and steroidal lactones. Choline, fatty acids, amino acids, and a variety of sugars are also found in the roots of ashwagandha. The essential oil responsible for its strong aroma has not been definitively characterized.

THE SCIENCE OF ASHWAGANDHA

Ashwagandha is often classified as an adaptogen, which means it helps to modify the harmful effects of stress on the body. Studies in animals have suggested that ashwagandha can limit the damage of free radicals through its antioxidant activity.[1, 2]

Ashwagandha has been shown to have a measurable effect on the immune system. It is capable of protecting the activity of immune cells that are subjected to chemicals that usually inhibit their function.[3, 4] This immune-protecting property of ashwagandha has been studied for the possible benefit of reducing the side effects of radiation and cancer chemotherapy treatments. The bone marrow of animals pretreated with ashwagandha that then receive radiation shows less suppression of production of infection-fighting white blood cells.[5] A similar protective effect was reported in animals taking ashwagandha prior to receiving a dose of the potent cancer-fighting drug cyclophosphamide.[6]

Ashwagandha may have a direct effect on limiting the growth of cancer cells. Extracts of ashwagandha may also increase the sensitivity of cancer cells to the effects of radiation therapy.[7] The combination of its ability to protect healthy cells while making cancerous ones more sus-ceptible to treatment suggests that ashwagandha may play an important role in modern cancer therapy. Further studies are needed to determine if this potential benefit can be realized in people.

One of the classic uses of ashwagandha is to calm mental turbulence. Some studies looking into the influence of ashwagandha on the brain have reported effects on GABA receptors, the site of action of tranquilizing drugs such as Valium and Ativan.[8] Other investigators have shown that the herb acts on acetylcholine receptors, known to be important in the processing of memory.[9] Studies on the relevancy of these laboratory findings to humans are limited. One report of men and women given daily doses of ashwagandha for forty days showed that those receiving the herb performed better on tests of logical thinking, problem solving, and reaction time than did a control group taking ginseng.[10] These reports suggest that the mind-tonic reputation of ashwagandha may be understood in scientific terms. More research is clearly warranted.

THE PRACTICAL USE OF ASHWAGANDHA

We use ashwagandha at the Chopra Center for its tonic and rejuvenative effects. With its beneficial influence on the nervous system, we commonly prescribe it for people who complain of fatigue, difficulty in concentrating, and a general sense of ungroundedness. Mixed with warm milk and taken before bed, ashwagandha is useful for people with insomnia and anxiety. It has a reputation in Ayurveda as a rejuvenative in conditions of nerve and muscle weakness. It is also used for men and women who are having trouble with fertility. Although it is sometimes recommended in India to strengthen pregnant women, we do not recommend nonculinary herbs or spices in pregnancy until safety and efficacy studies are performed.

In patients facing cancer, ashwagandha can be a valuable ally. As discussed above, it may have value during treatments but we more commonly recommend it in the recuperative phase as people are attempting to regain their energy and strength.

How to Use Ashwagandha

Several American herbal companies are now offering ashwagandha in doses of 300 to 500 milligrams. In some formulations the tablets are standardized to a specific dose of withanolides. The usual dose is 600 to 1000 milligrams twice daily. A tablet or teaspoon of powdered ashwagandha crushed in hot milk and sweetened with honey or sugar enhances its sedating qualities.

Ayurveda and Ashwagandha

Ashwagandha is a beneficial rejuvenating herb for both Vata and Kapha imbalances. Carrying the three tastes of bitter, astringent, and sweet, it can be a tonic for all three doshas, although because it is mildly heating it can slightly aggravate Pitta when taken in excess.

Precautions

Very large doses of ashwagandha have been reported to induce abortions in animals. Despite the lack of similar reports in human, ashwagandha should be avoided in pregnancy. Large doses may also cause mild digestive upset so it should be used cautiously in people with known peptic ulcer disease.

Circulatory/Respiratory	Detoxifier	Digestive	Immune Enhancer	Men's Health
			X	X
Metabolic	Nervine	Rejuvenative	Rheumatic	Women's Health
	X	X		

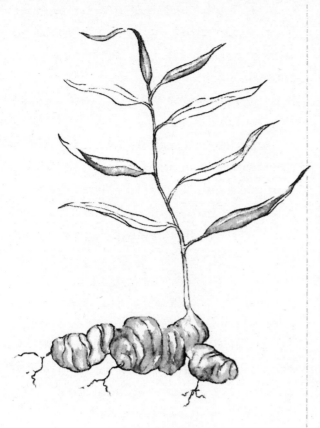

ZINGIBER OFFICINALE

FAMILIAR: **ginger**
LATIN: *Zingiber officinale*
SANSKRIT: andraka (fresh); sunthi (dry)

Known in Ayurveda as the universal remedy, ginger has been honored around the world and across time for its unique culinary and medicinal properties. From Confucius to Marco Polo to the Indian King Akbar, those who experienced the unique pungent flavor of ginger praised this powerful natural agent. Healers of medieval times traced the origins of ginger to the Garden of Eden, while, on the Indian subcontinent, references to this "king of spices" are found in the earliest myths. Known for its concentrated heating potency, ginger has been used across Asia and Africa to kindle the body's internal fire.

BOTANICAL AND PHYTOCHEMICAL INFORMATION

The ginger plant grows to about one meter high, but it is the underground rhizome that is prized for its spicy aromatic flavor and aroma. About 2 percent of the rootstock consists of a yellow volatile oil that contains a number of chemicals including camphene, zingiberine, and gingerol. The last of these, gingerol, appears to be responsible for ginger's pungent taste.

Originally from Asia, ginger is now widely cultivated throughout warm climatic regions, where its rhizomes are harvested before their first birthday. Ginger is used fresh, dried, and as a frequent ingredient in candies, chutneys, and preserves. Drying the root increases its irritant properties, but serious side effects have not been described.

THE SCIENCE OF GINGER

Ginger is best known for its effects on the digestive system. When taken internally, it stimulates the release of salivary enzymes and enhances stomach emptying. As a result, ginger has been used successfully to treat nausea and vomiting in a number of conditions. A study from England showed that ginger can prevent nausea after gynecological surgical procedures, although a more recent report from South Africa could not confirm this benefit.[1, 2] A Swiss study looked at ginger's efficacy in the treatment of seasickness and found it to be as useful as most medications commonly used, confirming an earlier report that showed ginger to be effective in motion sickness.[3, 4]

One of the most promising uses of ginger is in the treatment of morning sickness associated with pregnancy. Because of risks to the fetus, most drugs are diligently avoided during pregnancy. Gingerroot seems to offer a safe and effective option. Studies from Denmark found that almost three out of four pregnant women experienced some relief from their nausea without any limiting side effects.[5] The German Commission E has suggested that ginger be avoided in pregnancy owing to theoretical concerns, although no cases of ginger toxicity have yet been reported.

Considering its widespread usage without documented problems, ginger seems to be an acceptable antinausea substance when taken in normal doses.[6] Use only natural fresh gingerroot to gain maximal benefit with minimal risk.

Another potential use for ginger is in the treatment of nausea associated with cancer chemotherapy. In a recent animal study from India, ginger helped to stimulate the stomach to empty after a potent chemotherapy drug, cisplatin, was given.[7] Although there are many new effective antinausea drugs available to treat the side effects of cancer therapies, they are generally very expensive and carry side effects. In this study, ginger was found to be as effective as the most commonly used drug.

Ginger also has potentially beneficial effects on circulation. Animal studies suggest that ginger may help lower cholesterol levels and reduce the stickiness of platelets.[8, 9] A benefit that has been noted for thousands of years is ginger's ability to improve circulation. Both Chinese and Indian physicians prescribed ginger for people troubled by cold hands and feet, a remedy we have found consistently helpful at the Chopra Center.

THE PRACTICAL USE OF GINGER

Ginger is a beloved healing ally at the Chopra Center. We make fresh gingerroot tea continuously available to our guests and patients, encouraging them to sip three to four cups per day as part of their detoxification program. According to Ayurveda, ginger is one of the few medicinal substances that works on all three phases of gastrointestinal function: digestion, absorption, and elimination. We use ginger as part of our herbal apéritif, prepared by combining fresh gingerroot juice with equal parts water, lemon juice, and honey. An ounce taken at the start of a meal adds a spicy kick-start to the digestive process.

The juice can also be used for external purposes when added to a carrier oil and massaged into the sore spot. The essential volatile oil in ginger has a mild local heating effect. When applied to the skin for the treatment of rheumatic conditions, it stimulates local circulation, acting as a counterirritant. A ginger paste can also be applied directly to the head for the treatment of tension or migraine headaches. For sore muscles we recommend adding a few teaspoons of ginger powder to a hot bath before soaking.

Its pungent properties are also used to treat respiratory and circulatory problems. For people with cold hands and feet, drinking ginger tea or chewing on fresh or candied ginger can bring heat into the system. If you are feeling the onset of a cold, chew on fresh gingerroot to help clear your congested nasal passages.

If you are traveling on a boat or anticipating a turbulent plane ride, keep a piece of fresh ginger with you and nibble on it when your stomach feels queasy. If you are pregnant and experiencing morning sickness, chewing on a small piece of ginger may settle your delicate stomach.

How to Use Ginger

Ginger is now universally available. It can be found in almost every grocery store, where it can be purchased for less than twenty cents an ounce. It is readily obtainable as a ground, dried powder, and can be found as a candy in many Asian food markets.

Our recipe for ginger tea uses one teaspoon of grated root per one pint of hot water. If the tea is a little too pungent for you, try adding a teaspoon of shredded or chopped licorice root along with the ginger. When used as an externally applied substance, obtain the fresh juice by removing the outer fibrous layer and putting the inner part of the root through a juicer. Then mix equal parts of the ginger juice with a carrier oil such as almond or sesame, and massage into the sore muscle or joint. To relieve a migraine, mix a tablespoon of dry powder with a few drops of hot water until it is the consistency of a paste, then apply to your forehead and temples and sit in a warm bath.

AYURVEDA AND GINGER

From an Ayurvedic perspective, ginger's heating qualities make it useful for both Vata and Kapha disorders. Fresh ginger is better for Vata imbalances, as its moisture content does not aggravate the dryness of the Wind element. Dry ginger is good for Kapha accumulations, where both the heat and dryness can balance the wet coldness of Kapha, expressed in such conditions as sinus congestion and obesity.

PRECAUTIONS

If you are experiencing indigestion or heartburn, limit your internal use of ginger, as it can cause overheating. Combining ginger with licorice root can help to balance its Pitta-aggravating properties. Since ginger appears to have mild anti-platelet-forming effects, it should be used cautiously by people who are on prescribed blood thinners.

Circulatory/Respiratory	Detoxifier	Digestive	Immune Enhancer	Men's Health
X	X	X		
Metabolic	Nervine	Rejuvenative	Rheumatic	Women's Health
X	X		X	

8

Navigating the Herbal Forest

Throughout this book we have presented our view that herbal medicines are valuable components of a holistic health approach. During your exploration of the different botanical allies we have described, several important questions may have arisen in your mind. When discussing herbs, we commonly hear the following ones:

- How do I determine which herb I should take?
- Over what period of time should I take an herbal remedy?
- Is it beneficial to take several herbs together?
- Can I safely mix herbs and pharmaceutical drugs?
- What is the appropriate role of other, non-herbal nutritional supplements?

These are significant questions, and you will get many different answers depending upon the experience, background, and theoretical framework of the person you ask. Before offering you our responses, we again want to remind you to evaluate honestly the other important aspects of your life before expecting an herb to heal you. Take time each day to settle your mind through meditation. Commune with nature on a regular basis. Focus on eating a healthy, balanced diet with abundant fruits, vegetables, whole grains, and beans. Be sure to get enough rest. Minimize toxic substances, emotions, and relationships in your life. Only after you have addressed these essential elements of good health is it time to consider the appropriate use of herbal medicines. An herb is much more likely to be effective if your overall lifestyle is nurturing to your body, mind, and soul. So, without claiming that we have the definitive answers, we offer our responses to the questions posed above.

How Do I Determine Which Herb I Should Take?

We recommend beginning with a rasayana or rejuvenative herb if you are not facing a specific or serious health concern. A daily dose of ginseng or gotu kola can help raise your overall level of well-being. According to Ayurveda, the herbal tonic jam derived from amalaki (traditionally called Chavan Prash) can be taken by almost anyone, regardless of age or sex. Rejuvenative substances are designed to provide balanced herbal nutrition to enhance the body's natural resistance to illness. They are best considered subtle foods that provide an herbal foundation to strengthen mind-body integration.

If, after taking a general herbal tonic, you feel the specific need to enliven your masculine energy, consider adding ashwagandha or atmagupta to your diet. If you feel your feminine energy is lacking, try taking shatavari or black cohosh. A basic rejuvenative such as amalaki combined with ashwagandha or shatavari may be all you need to maintain optimal vitality.

Using an herb for a specific symptom or ailment requires sensitivity and awareness. We recommend that you first identify your primary health concern and choose one or two herbs that address your problem. Be certain that you are receiving a high-quality botanical agent, and take it as recommended. Although many herbal formulas contain dozens of components, be sure that you are receiving enough of any individual one to justify its inclusion. We generally do not encourage people to take more than a few supplements at a time. Be clear about your intended outcome, and tune in to your body's inner wisdom to see if you are achieving the effects you are seeking.

If, after an adequate period of time, you are not satisfied with the results, consider discontinuing the supplements you are taking and reevaluating the problem at another level. For example, if you have been dealing with recurrent viral infections, rather than trying other immune-enhancing herbs, consider going on a detoxification program for a couple of weeks to cleanse your system. Then add a rejuvenative herb to boost your body's immunity. The effective use of herbal medicines is more art than science, and the artistry requires that you regularly check in with your inner intelligence.

OVER WHAT PERIOD OF TIME SHOULD I TAKE AN HERBAL REMEDY?

If you are dealing with a chronic health concern, you may need to take an herb for at least a couple of months before you notice its benefit. We often see people who are simultaneously taking many different nutritional supplements, but have not allowed enough time with any substance to adequately assess its effects. If you are experiencing incomplete benefits, it may be helpful to increase the amount you are taking. In our experience the safest way to do this is to add another dose during the day. In other words, if your muscle ache is slightly reduced by taking guggulu twice daily, increase your intake to three times a day. It is important to remember that most herbs are subtle medicinal substances and need time to help your mind and body reestablish balance. Patience is an important virtue in healing.

It is also helpful to bear in mind that some herbs work best when taken on a continuous basis, and that others have a limited duration of efficacy. Echinacea is a good example of an herb that is best used for a short time during the early stages of a cold or flu, but loses its potency if taken regularly. Herbs that have an influence on the mind, such as kava kava or valerian, are also best used on an intermittent basis.

IS IT BENEFICIAL TO TAKE SEVERAL HERBS TOGETHER?

There is not a simple answer to this question. In many of the traditional medical systems, the combining of numerous herbs into a formula has been the rule. The classical texts of Ayurveda and traditional Chinese medicine expound the view that the blending of different herbs has a synergistic action and can minimize undesirable side effects. Modern medicine takes the opposite point of view, with an emphasis on standardized single chemicals. We take a middle road. Our experience has demonstrated that combining different herbs can balance and potentiate their efficacy. On the other hand, formulas that contain dozens of botanical constituents in subtherapeutic doses are unlikely to produce the desired effects. If you are taking a large number of nutritional supplements and you experience an adverse reaction, it is difficult to identify the responsible agent. We encourage you to gain as much information as possible about the herbal product you are taking and, to the extent possible, keep it simple.

Can I Safely Mix Herbs and Pharmaceutical Drugs?

The classical medical systems never addressed this question because synthesized drugs were not available at the time they were compiling their herbal formularies. We do not support the point of view that because herbs are "natural" they do not negatively interact with pharmacological medications. There are enough reports in the medical literature on adverse supplement/medication interactions to tread cautiously when mixing herbs with drugs. Calming herbs may potentiate the tranquilizing effects of drugs. Herbs that have a blood-thinning action may interfere with anticoagulant medications. How an herb is metabolized and eliminated from the body can influence the metabolism and elimination of drugs.

Our approach at the Chopra Center is to use herbs sparingly if a person is on a prescribed medication. If the possibility exists of eliminating a medicine and accomplishing similar benefits with a natural approach, we monitor the transition very carefully. We encourage you strongly to have an open and honest dialogue with your health-care provider before adding a medicinal herb or discontinuing any prescription medication. Do not risk your health through denial or wishful thinking. On the other hand, we believe it is a worthy goal to find the subtlest approach that can accomplish the intended outcome.

What Is the Appropriate Role of Other, Non-herbal Nutritional Supplements?

We envision a nutritional spectrum that spans the range from food on one end to drugs on the other. In between are supplements and herbs. As anyone who has recently walked into a health-food store is aware, there is an explosive growth in the nutriceutical world; dozens of new isolated substances are coming to market with a wide range of claimed health benefits. Nutritional derivatives including pycnogenols, coenzyme Q-10, grapeseed extract, green tea catechins, quercetin, MSM, blue-green algae, SAM-e, carnitine, and others are being consumed by increasing numbers of people. The research on many of these substances is often compelling, but it is difficult to know how to use them appropriately other than in a scattershot manner. In several of our vitamin and circulation formulas we have included these derivatives in combination with standard vitamins and minerals, because we believe the preliminary data warrants their inclusion. We view them as helping to supplement the nutritional value of food, but not as a substitute for good nutrition or for the appropriate use of herbal medicines.

Our recommendation for you is to do what we do—monitor the data. When we learn about a new supplement, we gather as much information as possible before adding it to our nutritional program. Research what is known, and determine whether its intended benefits are of particular value for you. Our general principle is "when in doubt, leave it out." Again, do not substitute the latest extracted agent for freshly prepared delicious meals.

NEW CONTEMPORARY MEDICINE

The evolutionary process moves in spirals. As our society circles back around to a more natural approach, we believe it is important to keep an open heart and mind, integrating the best of the old and the new. To us this means that whether an approach is ancient or modern does not, on it own, insure its significance. The only constant in life is change, and we must be open to a dynamic vision of healing if we are not to overlook potentially valuable approaches. On the other hand, in our exuberance to find the fountain of youth, we must temper our enthusiasm for every new promise with a mature, balanced assessment. Our goal is nothing short of perfect health. To this end, we hope that *The Chopra Center Herbal Handbook* provides you with a valuable map for this stage of your journey.

EPILOGUE

Wisdom traditions from time immemorial proclaim that the human body and the cosmic body are reflections of each other. The intelligence that orchestrates the activity of our minds and bodies is the same as that which orchestrates the activity of the universe.

When we look out at nature and see a plant, we normally do not say to ourselves, "This plant has a body and a mind." And yet the intelligence that is orchestrating the activity of the plant is the same as the intelligence within us. The environment is our extended body, and the plants and trees of this planet are aspects of ourselves. We are intimately and inseparably interconnected. We share the same raw materials—the same recycled earth, life force, mind, and spirit. The ancient sages declared that the inner intelligence of our bodies is the ultimate and supreme genius of nature, and mirrors the wisdom of the universe.

In the pages of this book you have gained a lot of information about how the body/mind of the herbal kingdom functions. When you read about the properties of herbs, you are learning about how the universe expresses itself in the botanical domain of awareness. When you ingest the herb, you are using the elements and forces in your extended body/mind—the world of plants—to correct the mistakes in your personal body/mind.

Knowledge and information are not synonymous. As we look at the great strides we have made in the biological sciences, we see that in many instances we have sacrificed wisdom for knowledge, knowledge for information, and information for data. The data is of minimal value if it does not lead to the expansion of wisdom. No book can replace your inner knowing, your inner genius, your inner wisdom. However, we hope this book will inspire you to explore those domains of awareness where you intuitively feel how to use the inner and outer resources of nature to enliven your healing process. Read this book carefully, over and over again. Study the traditional applications of the different herbs and formulas, but most important, listen to your body. Even as you make use of the suggestions in this book, become aware of the intuitive, wondrous, miraculous processes in your own body. At the same time, cultivate the awareness of what is happening in your subtle body—your emotions, feelings, memories, and desires.

In time you will begin to witness your self as you breathe, move, sit, eat, digest, metabolize, eliminate, and experience the world through your five senses. Creating balance in body and mind is the first step in healing, but health is more than the absence of disease. It is more than physical, emotional, and social well-being. It is more than fitness and vitality. Health is ultimately a higher state of consciousness.

Ayurveda reminds us that we are ripples of awareness in a vast ocean of con-sciousness. Every time we become imbalanced, even with a minor illness, it reflects a disruption in our harmonious relationship to the whole. The universe contains within its very nature the ability to reestablish balance. The cosmos is too grand, too powerful, and too intelligent to tolerate disruption for long. When we consciously participate in restoring our well-being to its ultimate level, we join in the cosmic dance. Health becomes more than just physical, emotional, and social fitness. It becomes the spontaneous fulfillment of desires. It becomes a domain of awareness in which there is magic, enthusiasm, and wonder. It becomes a state of personal transformation—a journey into healing. It becomes a journey toward God. Nothing less will provide the level of health we are all seeking. Nothing less will satisfy us.

NOTES

CHAPTER 1.
THE HERBAL RENAISSANCE

1. Eisenberg DM, Davis RB, et al. Trends in alternative medicine use in the United States, 1990–1997. *JAMA* 1998;280:1569–1575.
2. Elder NC, Gillcrist A, Minz R. Use of alternative health care by family practice patients. *Arch Fam Med* 1997;6:181–184.

CHAPTER 2.
A BRIEF TOUR THROUGH HERBAL HISTORY

1. Cragg GM. Paclitaxel (Taxol): a success story with valuable lessons for natural product drug discovery and development. *Med Res Rev.* 1998; 18:315–331.
2. King SR, Tempesta MS. From shaman to human clinical trials: the role of industry in ethnobotany, conservation and community reciprocity. In Ciba Foundation Symposium. *Ethnobotany and the Search for New Drugs.* Chichester, England: John Wiley & Sons. 1994;197–213.
3. Johnston B. One-third of nation's adults use herbal remedies: market estimated at $3.24 billion. *Herbal-Gram* 1997;40:49.
4. Eisenberg DM, Davis RB, et al. Trends in alternative medicine use in the United States, 1990–1997. *JAMA* 1998;280:1569–1575.
5. Le Bars PL, Katz MM, et al. A placebo-controlled, double-blind, randomized trial of an extract of Gingko biloba for dementia. North American EGb Study Group. *JAMA* 1997;278:1327–1332.
6. Hippius H. St Johns Wort (Hypericum perforatum) an herbal antidepressant. *Curr Med Res Opin* 1998; 14:171–184.
7. Blumenthal M (ed.). *The Complete German Commission E Monographs.* Boston: American Botanical Council. 1998.
8. Wetzel MS, Eisenberg DM, Kaptchuk TJ. Courses involving complementary and alternative medicine at US medical schools. *JAMA* 1998;280:784–787.

GENERAL REFERENCES

1. Anderson FJ. *An Illustrated History of the Herbals.* New York: Columbia University Press. 1977.
2. Artuso A. *Drugs of Natural Origin.* New York: The Pharmaceutical Products Press. 1997.
3. Leake CD. *An Historical Account of Pharmacology to the 20th Century.* Springfield, Illinois: Charles C. Thomas. 1975.

CHAPTER 3.
HOLISTICALLY HERBAL
General Ayurvedic References

1. Chopra D. *Perfect Health.* New York: Harmony Books, 1991.
2. Frawley D. *Ayurvedic Healing.* Salt Lake City: Passage Press, 1989.

3. Lad V. *Ayurveda: The Science of Self-Healing.* Wilmot, WI: Lotus Press, 1984.
4. Simon D. *The Wisdom of Healing.* New York: Harmony Books, 1997.

AROMATHERAPY REFERENCES

1. Davis P. *Aromatherapy An A–Z.* Essex, England: Saffron Walden, 1988.
2. Lawless J. *Aromatherapy and the Mind.* San Francisco: Thorsons, 1994.
3. Miller L, Miller B. *Ayurveda and Aromatherapy.* Twin Lakes, WI: Lotus Press, 1995.

CHAPTER 4.
SCIENCE-OF-LIFE HERBOLOGY

1. Bhishagratna KK (ed.). *The Sushruta Samhita.* Varanasi, India: Chowkhamba Sanskrit Series Office, 1981:361–362.

General Ayurvedic Herbal References

1. Dash B. *A Handbook of Ayurveda.* New Delhi: Concept Publishing, 1987.
2. Kapoor LD. *Handbook of Ayurvedic Medicinal Plants.* Boca Raton, FL: CRC Press, 1990.
3. Lad V, Frawley D. *The Yoga of Herbs.* Santa Fe: Lotus Press, 1986.

CHAPTER 5.
RESTORING BALANCE, CREATING HEALTH

1. Platel K, Srinivasan K. Influence of dietary spices or their active principles on digestive enzymes of small intestinal mucosa in rats. *International Journal Food Science Nutrition* 1996; 47:55–59.
2. Monograph: Piper methysticum (kava kava). *Alternat Med Rev* 1998;6:458–460.
3. Hippius H. St John's Wort (Hypericum perforatum)—an herbal antidepressant. *Curr Med Res Opin* 1998;14:171–84.
4. Hasenohrl RU, Nichau CH, et al. Anxiolytic-like effect of combined extracts of Zingiber officinale and Ginkgo biloba in the elevated plus-maze. *Pharmacol Biochem Behav* 1996;53: 271–275.
5. Hirata JD, Swiersz LM, et al. Does dong quai have estrogenic effects in postmenopausal women? A double-blind, placebo-controlled trial. *Fertil Steril* 1997;68:981–986.
6. Heymsfield SB, Allison DB, et al. Garcinia cambogia (hydroxycitric acid) as a potential antiobesity agent. *JAMA* 1998;280:1596–1600.
7. Sharma P. Caraka Samhita. Chaukhambha Orientalia, Varanasi, India, vol. II. 1983; page 4.
8. Kim HJ, Woo DS, et al. The relaxation effects of ginseng saponin in rabbit corporal smooth muscle: is it a nitric oxide donor? *Br J Urol* 1998;82:744–748.
9. Wilt TJ, A Ishani, et al. Saw palmetto extracts for treatment of benign prostatic hyperplasia. *JAMA* 1998;280:1604–1609.
10. Barclay TS, Tsourounis C, McCart GM. Glucosamine. *Ann Pharmacother* 1998; 32(5): 574–579.
11. Duwiejua M, Zeitlin IJ, et al. Anti-inflammatory activity of resins from some species of the plant family Burseraceae. *Planta Med* 1993;59:12–16.
12. Yoshida Y, Wang MQ, et al. Immunomodulating activity of Chinese medicinal herbs and Oldenlandia diffusa in particular. *Int J Immunopharmacol* 1997;19:359–370.
13. Kapil A, Sharma S. Immunopotentiating compounds from Tinospora cordifolia. *J Ethnopharmacol* 1997;58:89–95.
14. Luper S. A review of plants used in the treatment of liver disease. *Alternat Med Rev* 1998; 3:410–421.
15. Sharma H. *Freedom from Disease.* Veda Publishing, Toronto. 1993;39–172.
16. Isaacsohn JL, Moser M, et al. Garlic powder and plasma lipids and lipoproteins: a multi-

center, randomized, placebo-controlled trial. *Arch Intern Med* 1998;158:1189–94.

17. Mashour NH, Lin GO, Frishman WH. Herbal medicine for the treatment of cardiovascular disease. *Arch Intern Med* 1998;158: 2225–2234.

18. Dwivedi S and Agarwal MP. Anitanginal and cardioprotective effects of Terminalia arjuna, an indigenous drug, in coronary artery disease. *J Assoc Phys India.* 1994;42:287–289.

19. Miller LG. Herbal medicinals: selected clinical considerations focusing on known or potential drug-herb interactions. *Arch Intern Med* 1998; 158:2200–2211.

THE FORTY HERBS OF THE CHOPRA CENTER FORMULARY

ALLIUM SATIVUM/GARLIC

1. Warshafshy S, Kramer R, Sivak S. Effect of garlic on total serum cholesterol. *Ann Intern Med* 1993;119:599–605.

2. Silgay C, Neil A. Garlic as a lipid-lowering agent: a meta-analysis. *J R Coll Physicians London* 1994;28:2–8.

3. Steiner M, Khan AH, et al. A double-blind crossover study in moderately hypercholesterolemic men that compared the effect of aged garlic extract and placebo administration on blood lipids. *Am J Clin Nutr* 1996; 64:866–870.

4. Isaacsohn JL, Moser M, et al. Garlic powder and plasma lipids and lipoproteins: a multi-center, randomized, placebo-controlled trial. *Arch Intern Med* 1998;158:1189–1194.

5. Berthold HK, Sudhop T, von Bergmann K. Effect of a garlic oil preparation on serum lipoproteins and cholesterol metabolism: a randomized controlled trial. *JAMA* 1998; 270:1900–1902.

6. Bordia A, Verma SK, Srivastava KC. Effect of garlic (Allium sativum) on blood lipids, blood sugar, fibrinogen and fibrinolytic activity in patients with coronary artery disease. *Prostaglandins Leukot Essent Fatty Acids* 1998; 58:257–263.

7. Breithaupt-Grogler K, Ling M, et al. Protective effect of chronic garlic intake on elastic properties of aorta in the elderly. *Circulation* 1997;96:2649–2655.

8. Silagy CA, Neil HA. A meta-analysis of the effect of garlic on blood pressure. *J Hypertens* 1994;12:463–468.

9. Milner JA. Garlic: its anticarcinogenic and antitumorigenic properties. *Nutr Rev* 1996; 54:S82–S86.

10. Riggs DR, DeHaven JI, DL Lamm. Allium sativum (garlic) treatment for murine transitional cell carcinoma. *Cancer* 1997;79: 1987–1994.

11. Chen GW, Chung JG, et al. Effects of the garlic components diallyl sulfide and diallyl disulfide on arylamine N-acetyltransferase activity in human colon tumour cells. *Food Chem Toxicol* 1998;36:761–770.

12. Challier B, Perarnau JM, JF Viel. Garlic, onion and cereal fibre as protective factors for breast cancer: a French case-control study. *Eur J Epidemiol* 1998;14:737–747.

13. Dorant E, van den Brandt PA, et al. Garlic and its significance for the prevention of cancer in human: a critical view. *Br J Cancer* 1993;67:424–429.

14. Ledezma E, DeSousa L, et al. Efficacy of ajoene, an organosulphur derived from garlic, in the short-term therapy of tinea pedis. *Mycoses* 1996;39:393–395.

15. Abdullah TH. In vitro efficacy of a compound derived from garlic against Pneumocystis carinni. *J Nat Med Assoc* 1996;88: 694–704.

16. Sivam GP, Lampe JW, et al. Helicobacter pylori—in vitro susceptibility to garlic (Allium sativum) extract. *Nutr Cancer* 1997;27:118–121.

ALOE VERA/ALOE

1. Collins CE, Collins C. Roentgen dermatitis treated with fresh whole leaf in *Aloe vera. Am J Roentenol* 1935;33:396–397.
2. Chithra P, Sajithlal GB, Chandrakasan G. Influence of Aloe vera on collagen turnover in healing of dermal wounds in rats. *Indian J Exp Biol* 1998;36:896–901.
3. Davis RH, Leitner MG, et al. Antiinflammatory activity of Aloe vera against a spectrum of irritants. *J Am Podiatr Med Assoc* 1989;79:263–276.
4. Visuthikosol V, Chowchuen B, et al. Effect of aloe vera gel to healing of burn wound: a clinical and histologic study. *J Med Assoc Thai* 1995;78:403–409.
5. Syed TA, Ahmad SA, et al. Management of psoriasis with Aloe vera extract in a hydrophilic cream: a placebo-controlled, double-blind study. *Trop Med Int Health* 1996;1:505–509.
6. Heggers JP, Robson MC, et al. Experimental and clinical observations on frostbite. *Ann Emerg Med* 1987;16:1056–1062.
7. Shamaan NA, Kadie KA, et al. Vitamin C and aloe vera supplementation protects from chemical hepatocarcinogenesis in the rat. *Nutrition* 1998;14:846–852.
8. Robinson M. Medical therapy of inflammatory bowel disease for the 21st century. *Eur J Surg Supl* 1998;(582):90–98.
9. Dykman KD, Tone C, et al. The effects of nutritional supplements on the symptoms of fibromyalgia and chronic fatigue syndrome. *Integr Physiol Behav Sci* 1998;33:61–71.
10. Blitz JJ, Smith JW, Gerard JR. *Aloe vera* gel in peptic ulcer therapy: preliminary report. *J Am Osteo Soc* 1963;62:731–735.

ANDROGRAPHIS PANICULATA/INDIAN GENTIAN

1. Choudhury BR, Poddar MK. Andrographolide and kalmegh (Andrographis paniculata) extract: in vivo and in vitro effect on heaptic lipid peroxidation. *Methods Find Exp Clin Pharmacol* 1984;6:481–485.
2. Melchior J. Controlled clinical study of standardized Andrographis panniculata extract in common cold—a pilot trial. *Phytomedicine* 1996/97;3:314–318.
3. Puri A, Saxena R, et al. Immunostimulant agents from Andrographis paniculata. *J Nat Prod* 1993;56:995–999.
4. Leelarasamee A, Trakulsomboon S, Sittisomwong N. Undetectable antibacterial activity of Andrographis paniculata (Burma) wall. Ex ness. *J Med Assoc Thai* 1990;73:299–304.
5. Najib Nik A Rahman N, Furuta T, et al. Antimalarial activity of extracts of Malayasian medicinal plants. *J Ethnopharmacol* 1999;64:249–254.
6. Dutta A, Sukul NC. Filaricidal properties of a wild herb, Andrographis paniculata. *J Helminthol* 1982;56:81–84.
7. Chang RS, Ding L, et al. Dehydroandrographolide succinic acid monester as an inhibitor against the human immunodeficiency virus. *Proc Soc Exp Biol Med* 1991;197:59–66.
8. Thamlitikul V, Dechatiwongse T, et al. Efficacy of Andrographis paniculata, Nees for pharyngotonsillitis in adults. *J Med Assoc Thai* 1991;74:437–442.
9. Muangman V, Visehsindh V, et al. The usage of Andrographis paniculata following extracorporeal shock wave lithotripsy (ESWL). *J Med Assoc Thai* 1995;78:310–313.
10. No authors listed. Paracelsian announces preliminary results of safety study show AndroVir well tolerated with decreases in HIV viral load and rapid increases in CD4 positive

cells. Access via: *www.aegis.com/news/pr/1996/PR961224.html*

11. Zhang C, Kuroyangi M, Tan BK. Cardiovascular activity of 14-deoxy-11,12-didehydroandrographolide in the anaesthetised rat and isolated right atria. *Pharmacol Res* 1998;38:413–417.

12. Guo Z, Zhao H, Fu L. Protective effects of API0134 on myocardial ischemia and reperfusion injury. *J Tongji Med Univ* 1996;16:193–197.

13. Amroyan E, Gabrielian E, et al. Inhibitory effect of andrographolide from Andrographis paniculata on PAF-induced platelet aggregation. *Phytomedicine* 1999;6:27–31.

14. Zhang YZ, Tang JZ, Zhang YJ. Study of Andrographis paniculata extracts on antiplatelet aggregation and release reaction and its mechanism. *Chung Kuo Chung His I Chieh Ho Tsa Chih* 1994;14:28–30.

15. Wang DW, Zhao HY. Experimental studies on prevention of atherosclerosis arterial stenosis and restenosis after angioplasty with Andrographis paniculata Nees and fish oil. *J Tongji Med Univ* 1993;13:193–198.

16. Kapil A, Koul IB, et al. Antihepatotoxic effects of major diterpenoid constituents of Andrographis paniculata. *Biochem Pharmacol* 1993;46:182–185.

17. Rana AC, Avadhoot Y. Hepatoprotective effects of Andrographis paniculata against carbon tetrachloride-induced liver damage. *Arch Pharm Res* 1991;14:93–95.

18. Visen PK, Shukla B, et al. Andrographolide protects rat hepatocytes against paracetamol-induced damage. *J Ethnopharmacol* 1993;40:131–136.

19. Shukla B, Visen PK, et al. Choleretic effect of andrographolide in rats and guinea pigs. *Planta Med* 1992;58:146–149.

20. See note 10 above.

*ASPARAGUS RACEMOSUS/*SHATAVARI

1. Joglekar GV, Ahuja RH, Balwani JH. Galactogogue effect of Asparagus racemosus. Preliminary communication. *Indian Med J* 1967;61:165.

2. Sabnis PB, Gaitonde BB, Jetmalani M. Effects of alcoholic extracts of Asparagus racemosus on mammary glands of rats. *Indian J Exp Biol* 1968;6:55–57.

3. Sharma S, Ramji S, et al. Randomized controlled trial of Asparagus racemosus (Shatavari) as a lactogogue in lactational inadequacy. *Indian Pediatr* 1996;33:675–677.

4. Dalvi SS, Nadkarni PM, Gupta KC. Effect of Asparagus racemosus (Shatavari) on gastric emptying time in normal healthy volunteers. *J Postgrad Med* 1990;36:91–4.

5. Rege NN, Dahanukar SA. Quantitation of microbicidal activity of mononuclear phagocytes: an in vitro technique. *J Postgrad Med* 1993;39:22–25.

6. Dhuley JN. Effect of some Indian herbs on macrophage functions in ochratoxin A–treated mice. *J Ethnopharmacol* 1997;58:15–20.

7. Thatte UM, Dahanukar SA. Comparative study of immunomodulating activity of Indian medicinal plants, lithium carbonate and glucan. *Methods Find Exp Clin Pharmacol* 1988;10:639–644.

8. Rege NN, Nazareth HM, et al. Immunotherapeutic modulation of intraperitoneal adhesions by Asparagus racemosus. *J Postgrad Med* 1989;35:199–203.

*ASTRAGALUS MEMBRANACEUS/*ASTRAGALUS

1. Chu DT, Wong WL, Mavligit GM. Immunotherapy with Chinese medicinal herbs. II. Reversal of cyclophsoaminde-induced immune suppression by administration of fractionated Astragalus membranaceus in vivo. *J Clin Lab Immunol* 1988;25:125–129.

2. Zhao KS, Mancini C, Doria G. Enhancement of the immune response in mice by Astragalus membranaceus extracts. *Immunopharmacology* 1990;20:224–233.

3. Lau BH, Ruckle HC, et al. Chinese medicinal herbs inhibit growth of murine renal cell carcinoma. *Cancer Biother* 1994;9:153–161.

4. Peng T, Yang Y, et al. The inhibitory effect of astragalus membranaceus on coxsackie B-3 virus RNA replication. *Chin Med Sci J* 1956;10:146–150.

5. Sun Y, Hersh EM, et al. Preliminary observations on the effects of the Chinese medicinal herbs Astragalus membranaceus and Ligustrum lucidum on lymphocyte blastogenic responses. *J Biol Response Mod* 1983;2:227–237.

6. Chu DT, Wong WL, Mavligit GM. Immunotherapy with Chinese medicinal herbs. I. Immune restoration of local xenogeneic graft-versus-host reaction in cancer patients by fractionated Astragalus membranaceus in vitro. *J Clin Lab Immunol* 1988;25:119–123.

7. Chu DT, Lepe-Zuniga J, et al. Fractionated extract of Astragalus membranaceus, a Chinese medicinal herb, potentiates LAK cell cytotoxicity by a low dose of recombinant interleukin-2. *J Clin Lab Immunol* 1988;26:183–187.

8. Cha RJ, Seng DW, Chang QS. Non-surgical treatment of small cell lung cancer with chemo-radio-immunotherapy and traditional Chinese medicine. *Chung Hua Nei Ko Tsa Chih* 1994;33:462–466.

9. Zhao XZ. Effects of Astragalus membranaceus and Tripterygium hypoglancum on natural killer cell activity of peripheral blood mononuclear cells in systemic lupus erythematosus. *Chung Kuo Chung Hsi I Chieh Ho Tsa Chih* 1992;12:669–671.

10. Huang ZQ, Qin NP, Ye W. Effect of Astragalus membranaceus on T-lymphocyte subsets in patients with viral myocarditis. *Chung Kuo Chung Hsi I Chieh Ho Tsa Chih* 1995;15:328–330.

11. Li SQ, Yuan RX, Gao H. Clinical observation on the treatment of ischemic heart disease with Astragalus membranaceus. *Chung Kuo Chung Hsi I Chieh Ho Tsa Chih* 1995;15:77–80.

12. Lei ZY, Qin H, Liao JZ. Action of Astragalus membranaceus on left ventricular function of angina pectoris. *Chung Kuo Chung Hsi I Chieh Ho Tsa Chih* 1994;14:199–202.

13. Hong CY, Lo YC, et al. Astragalus membranaceus and Polygonum multiflorum protect rat heart mitochondria against lipid peroxidation. *Am J Chin Med* 1994;22:63–70.

14. Hong HX, Qin WC, Huang LS. Memory-improving effect of aqueous extract of Astragalus membranaceus (Fisch,) Bge. *Chung Kuo Chung Yao Tsa Chih* 1994;19:687–688.

15. Hong CY, Ku J, Wu P. Astragalus membranaceus stimulates human sperm motility in vitro. *Am J Chin Med* 1992;20:289–294.

16. Zhang ZL, Wen QZ, Liu CX. Hepatoprotective effects of astragalus root. *J Ethnopharmacol* 1990;30:145–159.

AZADIRACHTA INDICA/NEEM

1. Fabry W, Okemo PO, Ansorg R. Antibacterial activity of East African medicinal plants. *J Ethnopharmacol* 1998;60:79–84.

2. Fabry W, Okemo P, Ansorg R. Fungistatic and fungicidal activity of east African medicinal plants. *Mycoses* 1996;39:67–70.

3. Ray A, Banerjee BD, Sen P. Modulation of humoral and cell-meditated immune responses by Azadirachta indica (Neem) in mice. *Ind J Exp Biol* 1996;34:698–701.

4. Wolinsky LE, Mania S et al. The inhibiting effect of aqueous Azadirachta indica (Neem) extract upon bacterial properties influencing in vitro plaque formation. *J Dent Res* 1996;75:816–822.

5. Charles V, Charles SX. The use and efficacy of Azadirachta indica ADR ('Neem') and Curcuma longa ('Turmeric') in scabies. A pilot study. *Trop Geogr Med* 1992;44:178–181.

6. Chattopadhyay RR. Possible biochemical modes of anti-inflammatory action of Azadirachta indica A. Juss. in rats. *Indian J Exp Biol* 1998;36:418–420.

7. Khanna N, Goswami M, et al. Antinociceptive action of Azadirachta indica (neem) in mice: possible mechanisms involved. *Indian J Exp Biol* 1995;33:848–850.

8. Jaiswal Ak, Bhattacharya SK, Acharya SB. Anxiolytic activity of Azadirachta indica leaf extract in rats. *Indian J Exp Biol* 1994;32:489–491.

9. Garg GP, Nigam SK, Ogle CW. The gastric antiulcer effects of the leaves of the neem tree. *Planta Med* 1993;59:215–217.

10. Chattopadhyay RR. Possible mechanism of antihyperglycemic effect of Azadirachta indica leaf extract. Part IV. *Gen Pharmacol* 1996;27:431–434.

11. Garg S, Talwar GP, Upadhyay SN. Immunocontraceptive activity guided fractionation and characterization of active constituents of neem (Azadirachta indica) seed extracts. *J Ethnopharmacol* 1998;60:235–246.

12. Mukherjee S, Lohiya NK, et al. Purified neem (Azadirachta indica) seed extracts (Praneem) abrogate pregnancy in primates. *Contraception* 1996;53:375–378.

BOSWELLIA SERRATA/BOSWELLIN

1. Sharma ML, Bani S, et al. Anti-arthritic activity of boswellic acid in bovine serum albumin-induced arthritis. *Indian J Immunopharmac* 1989;6:647–652.

2. Safayhi H, Mack T, et al. Boswellic acids: novel, specific nonredox inhibitors of 5-lipoxygenase. *J Pharmacol Exp Ther* 1992;261:1143–1146.

3. Ammon HPT, Safayhi H, et al. Mechanisms of anti-inflammatory actions of curcurmine and boswellic acids. *J Ethnopharmacol* 1993;38:113–119.

4. Wildfeuer A, Neu IS, et al. Effects of boswellic acids extracted from a herbal medicine on the biosynthesis of leukotrienes and the course of experimental autoimmune encephalomyelitis. *Arzneimettelforschung* 1998;48:668–674.

5. Ammon HP, Mack T, et al. Inhibition of leukotriene B4 formation in rat peritoneal neutrophils by an ethanolic extract of the gum resin exudate of Boswellia serrata. *Planta Med* 1991;57:203–207.

6. Gupta I, Gupta V, et al. Effects of Boswellia serrata gum resin in patients with bronchial asthma: results of a double-blind, placebo-controlled, 6-week clinical study. *Eur J Med Res* 1998;17:511–514.

7. Reddy GK, Chandrakasan G, Dhar SC. Studies on the metabolism of glycosaminoglycans under the influence of new herbal anti-inflammatory agents. *Biochem Phamracol* 1989;38:3527–3534.

8. Kulkarni RR, Patki PS, et al. Treatment of osteoarthritis with a herbomineral formulation: a double-blind, placebo-controlled, crossover study. *J Ethnopharmacol* 1991;33:91–95.

9. Sander O, Herborn G, Rau R. Is H15 (resin extract of Boswellia serrata, "incense") a useful supplement to established drug therapy of chronic polyarthritis? Results of a double-blind pilot study. *Z Rheumatol* 1998;57:11–16.

10. Gupta I, Parihar A, et al. Effects of Boswellia serrata gum resin in patients with ulcerative colitis. *Eur J Med Res* 1997;2:37–43.

CAMELLIA SINENSIS/TEA

1. Paganga G, Miller N, Rice-Evans CA. The polyphenolic content of fruit and vegetables

and their antioxidant activities. What does a serving constitute? *Free Radic Res* 1999;30: 153–162.

2. Serafini M, Ghiselli A, Ferro-Luzzi A. In vivo antioxidant effect of green and black tea in man. *Eur J Clin Nutr* 1996;50:28–32.

3. Zhu M, Gong Y, Yang Z. Protective effect of tea on immune function in mice. *Chung Hua Yu Fang I Hseuh Tsa Chih* 1998;32:250–274.

4. Han C. Screening of anticarinogenic ingredients in tea polyphenols. *Cancer Lett* 1997;114: 153–158.

5. Conney AH, Lu Y, et al. Inhibitory effect of green and black tea on tumor growth. *Proc Soc Exp Biol Med* 1999;220:229–233.

6. Nakachi K, Suemasu K, et al. Influence of drinking green tea on breast cancer malignancy among Japanese patients. *Jpn J Cancer Res* 1998;89:254–261.

7. Gupta S, Ahmad N, Mukhtar H. Prostate cancer chemoprevention by green tea. *Semin Urol Oncol* 1999;17:70–76.

8. Kohlmeier L, Weterings KG, et al. Tea and cancer prevention: an evaluation of the epidemologic literature. *Nutr Cancer* 1997;27: 1–13.

9. Matsumoto N, Okushio K, Hara Y. Effect of black tea polyphenols on plasma lipidsin cholesterol-fed rats. *J Nutr Sci Vitaminol (Tokyo)* 1998;44:337–342.

10. Chan PT, Fong WP, et al. Jasmine green tea epicatechins are hypolipidemic in hamsters (Mesocricetus auratus) fed a high fat diet. *J Nutr* 1999;129:1094–1101.

11. Van het Hof KH, Wiseman SA, et al. Plasma and lipoprotein levels of tea catechins following repeated tea consumption. *Proc Soc Exp Biol Med* 1999;220:203–209.

12. Stensvold I, Tverdal A, et al. Tea consumption relationship to cholesterol, blood pressure and coronary and total mortality. *Prev Med* 1992;21:546–553.

13. Hollman PC, Feskens EJ, Katan MB. Tea flavonols in cardiovascular and cancer epidemology. *Proc Soc Exp Biol Med* 1999;220: 198–202.

14. Sadakata S, Fukao A, Hisamichi S. Mortality among female practitioners of Chanoyu (Japanese "tea-ceremony"). *Tohoku J Exp Med* 1992;166:475–477.

15. Hertog MG, Sweetman PM, et al. Antioxidant flavonols and ischemic heart disease in a Welsh population of men: the Caerphilly Study. *Am J Clin Nutr* 1997;65:1489–1494.

16. Otake S, Makimura M, et al. Anticaries effects of polyphenolic compounds from Japanese green tea. *Caries Res* 1991;25:438–443.

17. Han LK, Takaku T, et al. Anti-obesity action of oolong tea. *Int J Obes Relat Metab Disord* 1999;23:98–105.

18. Alic M. Green tea for remission maintenance in Crohn's disease? *Am J Gastroenterol* 1999;94:1710–1711.

19. Aizaki T, Osaka M, et al. Hypokalemia with syncope caused by habitual drinking of oolong tea. *Intern Med* 1999;38:252–256.

20. Taylor JR, Wilt VM. Probably antagonism of warfarin by green tea. *Ann Pharmacother* 1999;33:426–428.

CASSIA ANGUSTIFOLIA/SENNA

1. Franz G. The senna drug and its chemistry. *Pharmacology* 1993;47 (Suppl. 1):2–6.

2. Beubler E, Schirgi-Degen A. Serotonin antagonists inhibit sennoside-induced fluid secretion and diarrhea. *Pharmacology* 1993;47 (Suppl. 1):64–69.

3. Passmore AP, Wilson-Davies K, et al. Chronic constipation in long stay elderly patients: a comparison of lactulose and a senna-fiber combination. *BMJ* 1993;307:1425–1426.

4. Kinnumen O, Winblad I, et al. Safety and efficacy of a bulk laxative containing senna versus lactulose in the treatment of chronic

constipation in geriatric patients. *Pharmacology* 1993;47 (Suppl. 1):253–255.

5. Cameron JC. Constipation related to narcotic therapy. A protocol for nurses and patients. *Cancer Nurs* 1992;15:372–377.

6. Sykes NP. A volunteer model for the comparison of laxatives in opioid-related constipation. *J Pain Symptom Manage* 1996;11:363–369.

7. Corman ML. Management of postoperative constipation in anorectal surgery. *Dis Colon Rectum* 1979;22:149–151.

8. Shelton MG. Standardized senna in the management of constipation in the puerperium: a clinical trial. *S Afr Med J* 1980;57:78–80.

9. Valverde A, Hay JM, et al. Senna vs polyethylene glycol for mechanical preparation the evening before elective colonic or rectal resection: a multicenter controlled trial. *Arch Surg* 1999;134:514–519.

10. No author listed. Senna and habituation. *Pharmacology* 1992;44(Suppl. 1):30–32.

11. Haward LRC, Hughes-Roberts HE. The treatment of constipation in mental hospitals. *Gut* 1962;3:85–90.

12. Smith CW, Evans PR. Bowel motility. A problem in institutionalized geriatric care. *Geriatrics* 1961;16:189–192.

13. el-Saadany SS, el-Massry RA, et al. The biochemical role and hypocholesterolaemic potential of the legume Cassia fistula in hypercholesterolaemic rats. *Nahrung* 1991;35:897–815.

14. Malterud KE, Farbrot TL, et al. Antioxidant and radical scavenging effects of anthraquinones and anthrones. *Pharmacology* 1993;47 (suppl. 1):77–85.

15. Sydiskis RJ, Owen DG, et al. Inactivation of enveloped viruses by anthraquinones extracted from plants. *Antimicrob Agents Chemother* 1991;35:2463–2466.

16. Perumal Samy R, Ignacimuthu S, Sen A. Screening of 34 Indian medicinal plants for antibacterial properties. *J Ethnopharmacol* 1998;62:173–182.

17. Joo JS, Ehrenpreis ED, et al. Alterations in colonic anatomy induced by chronic stimulating laxatives: the cathartic colon revisited. *J Clin Gastroenterol* 1998;26:283–286.

18. Brusick D, Mengs U. Assessment of the genotoxic risk from laxative senna products. *Environ Mol Mutagen* 1997;29:1–9.

19. Gattuso JM, Kamm MA. Adverse effects of drugs used in the management of constipation and diarrhoea. *Drug Saf* 1994;10: 47–65.

20. Hagemann TM. Gastrointestinal medication and breastfeeding. *J Hum Lact* 1998;14: 259–262.

21. Faber P, Strenge-Hesse A. Relevance of rhein excretion into breast milk. *Pharmacology* 1988;36 (Suppl. 1):212–220.

CENTELLA ASIATICA/GOTU KOLA

1. Sunilkumar, Parameshwaraiah S, Shivakumar HG. Evaluation of topical formulations of aqueous extract of Centella asiatica on open wounds in rats. *Indian J Exp Biol* 1998;36:569–572.

2. Belcaro GV, Rulo A, Grimaldi R. Capillary filtration and ankle edema in patients with venous hypertension treated with TTFCA. *Angiology* 1990;41:12–18.

3. Appa Rao MVR, Srinvasan KK, Koteswara RTL. The effect of *Centella asiatica* on the general mental ability of mentally retarded children. *Ind J Psychiatry* 1977;19:54–59.

4. Tripathi YB, Chaurasia S, et al. Bacopa monniera Linn. as an antioxidant: mechanism of action. *Indian J Exp Biol* 1996;34: 523–526.

5. Singh HK, Dhawan BN. Effect of Bacopa monniera Linn. (brahmi) extract on avoidance responses in rat. *J Ethnopharmacol* 1982;5:205–214.

CIMICIFUGA RACEMOSA/BLACK COHOSH

1. Macht DI, Cook HM. A pharmacological note on cimicifuga. *J Am Pharm Assoc* 1932;21: 324–330.
2. Stolze H. The other way to treat symptoms of menopause. *Der Kassenarzt* 1983;23:39–41.
3. Daiber W. Menopause symptoms: success without hormones. *Arztliche Praxis* 1983;35: 1946–1947.
4. Vorberg G. Treatment of menopause symptoms. *Zeitschrift fur Allgemeinmedizin* 1984; 60:626–629.
5. Stoll W. Phytotherapy influences atrophic vaginal epithelium, *Therapeuticon* 1987;1:23–31.
6. Petho A. Menopause symptoms: Is it possible to switch from hormone treatment to a botanical gynecologicum? *Arztliche Praxis* 1987;47: 1551–1553.
7. Duker EM, Kopanski L, et al. Effects of extracts from Cimicifuga racemosa on gonadotropin release in menopausal women and ovariectomized rats. *Planta Med* 1991; 57:420–424.
8. Einer-Jensen N, Zhao J, et al. Cimicifuga and Melbrosia lack oestrogenic effects in mice and rats. *Maturitas* 1996;25:149–153.
9. Li JX, Kadota S, et al. Effects of Cimicifuga rhizoma on serum calcium and phosphate levels in low calcium dietary rats and on bone mineral density in ovariectomized rats. *Phytomedicine* 1997/97;3:379–385.
10. Lieberman S. A review of the effectiveness of Cimicifuga racemosa (Black cohosh) for the symptoms of menopause. *J Women's Health* 1998;7:525–529.
11. Genazzani E, Sorrentino L. Vascular action of acteina: active constituent of actaea racemosa L. *Nature* 1962;194:544–545.
12. Benoit PS, Fong HHS, et al. Biological and phytochemical evaluation of plants. XIV. Anti-inflammatory evaluation of 163 species. *Lloydia* 1976;39:160–171.
13. Farnsworth NR, Segelman AB. Hypoglycemic plants. *Till and Tile* 1971;57:52–56.

COLEUS FORSKOHLII/FORSKOLIN

1. Yanagihara H, Sakata R, et al. Rapid analysis of small samples containing forskolin using monoclonal antibodies. *Planta Med* 1996;62: 169–172.
2. Seamon KB, Padgett W, Daly JW. Forskolin: unique diterpene activator of adenylated cyclase in membranes and in intact cells. *Proc Natl Acad Sci* 1981;78:3363–3367.
3. Dubey MP, Srimal RC, et al. Pharmacological studies on coleonol, a hypotensive diterpene from Coleus forskohlii. *J Ethnopharmacol* 1981; 3:1–13.
4. Marone G, Columbo M, et al. Inhibition of IgE-mediated release of histamine and peptide leukotriene from human basophils and mast cells by forskolin. *Biochem Pharmacol* 1987;36:13–20.
5. Lindner E, Dohadwalla AN, Bhattacharya BK. Positive intoropic and blood pressure lowering activity of a diterpene derivative isolated from coleus forskohlii: forskolin. *Arzneim Forsch* 1978;28:284–289.
6. Kramer W, Thormann J, et al. Effects of forskolin on left ventricular function in dilated cardiomyopathy. *Arzneim Forsch* 1987; 37:364–367.
7. Agarwal KC, Zielinski BA, Maitra RS. Significance of plasma adenosine in the antiplatelet activity of forskolin: potentiation by dipyridamole and dilazep. *Thrmob Haemost* 1989;61:106–110.
8. Tsukawaki M, Suzuki K, et al. Relaxant effects of forskolin on guinea pig trachea smooth muscle. *Lung* 1987;165: 225–237.
9. Kreutner W, Chapman RW, et al. Bronchodilator and antiallergy activity of forskolin. *Eur J Pharmacol* 1985;111:1–8.

10. Bauer K, Dietersdorfer F, et al. Pharmacodynamic effects of inhaled dry powder formulations of fenoerol and colforsin in asthma. *Clin Pharmacol Ther* 1993;53:76–83.

11. Lichey J, Freidrich T, et al. Effect of forskolin on methacholine-induced bronchostriciton in extrinsic asthmatics. *Lancet* 1984;ii:167.

12. Kaik G, Witte PU. Protective effect of forskolin in acetylcholine provocation in healthy probands. Comparison of 2 doses with fenoterol and placebo. *Wien Med Wochenschr* 1986;136:637–641.

13. Caprioli J, Sears M, et al. Forskolin lowers intraocular pressure by reducing aqueous inflow. *Invest Ophthalmol Vis Sci* 1984;25:268–277.

14. Seto C, Eguchi S, et al. Acute effects of topical forskolin on aquesous humor dynamics in man. *Jap J Ophthalmol* 1986;30:238–244.

15. Meyer BH, Stulting AA, et al. The effects of forskolin eye drops on intraocular pressure. *S Afr Med J* 1987;71:570–571.

16. Podos SM, Camras CB, Serle JB. Experimental compounds to lower intracocular pressure. *Aust NZ J Ophthalmol* 1989;17:129–135.

17. Mulhall JP, Daller M, et al. Intrcavernosal forskolin: role in management of vasculogenic impotence resistant to standard 3-agent pharmacotherapy. *J Urol* 1997;158:1742–1759.

18. Wachtel H, Loschmann PA. Effects of forskolin and cyclic nucleotides in animal models predictive of antidepressant activity: interaction with rolipram. *Psychopharmacol* 1986;90:430–435.

19. Agarwal KC, Parks RE. Forskolin: a potential antimetastatic agent. *Int J Cancer* 1983; 15:801–804.

COMMIPHORA MUKUL/GUGGULU

1. Satyavati GV, Dwarakanath C, Tripathi SN. Experimental studies of the hypocholesterolemic effect of *Commiphora mukul. Ind J Med Res* 1969;57:1950–1962.

2. Singh RB, Niaz MA, Ghosh S. Hypolipidemic and antioxidant effects of Commiphora mukul as an adjunct to dietary therapy in patents with hypercholesterolemia. *Cardiovasc Drugs Ther* 1994;8:659–664.

3. Nityanand S, Srivastava JS, Asthana OP. Clinical trials with gugulipid. A new hypolipidaemic agent. *J Assoc Physicians India* 1989;37:323–328.

4. Mester L, Mester M, Nityanand S. Inhibition of platelet aggregation by "guggulu" steroids. *Planta Med* 1979;37:367–369.

5. Sharma JN, Sharma JN. Comparison of the anti-inflammatory activity of Commiphora mukul (an indigenous drug) with those of phenylbutazone and ibuprofen in experimental arthritis induced by mycobacterial adjuvant. *Arzneimittelforschung* 1977;27: 1455–1457.

6. Thappa DM, Dogra J. Nodulocystic acne: oral gugulipid versus tetracycline. *J Dermatol* 1994;21:729–731.

CRATAEGUS OXYACANTHA/HAWTHORN

1. Maffei Facino R, Carini M, et al. Free radical scavenging action and anti-enzyme activities of procyanidines from Vitis vinifera. *Arzneimittelforschung* 1994;44:592–601.

2. Uchida S, Ikara N, et al. Inhibiting effects of condensed tannins on angiotensin converting enzyme. *Jap J Pharmacol* 1987;43:242–245.

3. Shanthi S, Parasakthy K, et al. Hypolipidemic activity of tincture of Crataegus in rats. *Indian J Biochem Biophys* 1994;31:143–146.

4. Gabor M. Pharmacologic effects of flavonoids on blood vessels. *Angiologica* 1972;9:355–74.

5. al Makdessi, Sweidan H, et al. Myocardial protection by pretreatment with Crataegus oxyacantha: an assessment by means of the release of lactate dehydrogenase by the ischemic and reperfused Langendorff heart. *Arzneimittelforschung* 1996;46:25–27.

6. al Makdessi S, Sweidan H, et al. Protective effect of Crataegus oxyacantha against reperfusion arrhythmias after global no-flow ischemia in the rat heart. *Basic Res Cardiol* 1999;94:71–77.

7. Chatterjee SS, Koch E, et al. In vitro and in vivo investigations on the cardioprotective effects of oligomeric procyanidins in a Crataegus extract from leaves with flowers. *Arzneimittelforschung* 1997;47:821–825.

8. Blseken R. Crataegus in cardiology. *Fortschr Med* 1992;110:290–292.

9. Krzeminski T, Chatterjee SS. Ischemia and early reperfusion induced arrhythmias: beneficial effects of an extract of Crataegus oxyacantha L. *Pharm Pharmacol Lett* 1993;3: 345–348.

10. Schmidt U, Kuhn U, et al. Efficacy of hawthorn (Crataegus) preparation L1 132 in 78 patients with chronic congestive heart failure defined as NYHA functional class II. *Phytomedicine* 1994;1:17–24.

11. Weikl A, Assmus KD, et al. Crataegus special extract WS 1442: assessment of objective effectiveness in patients with heart failure. *Fortschr Med* 1996;114:291–296.

12. Ammon HP, Handel M. Crataegus, toxicology and pharmacology—Parts I, II, III. *Planta Medica* 1981;43:105–120, 209–239, 313–322.

Curcurma longa/Turmeric

1. Shalani VK, Srinivas L. Lipid peroxide induced DNA damage: protection by turmeric (Cucurma longa). *Free Radical Biol Med* 1991; 77:3–10.

2. Rafatullah S, Tariq M, et al. Evaluation of turmeric (Curcuma longa) for gastric and duodenal antiulcer activity in rats. *J Enthopharmacol* 1990;29:25–34.

3. Deshpande UR, Gadre SG, et al. Protective effect of turmeric (Curcuma longa L.) extract on carbon tetrachloride–induced liver damage in rats. *Indian J Exp Biol* 1998;36:573–577.

4. Dixit VP, Jain P, Joshi SC. Hypolipidaemic effects of Curcuma longa L. and Nardostachys jatamansi, DC in triton-induced hyperlipidaemic rats. *Indian J Physiol Pharmacol* 1988;32:299–403.

5. Srivastava KC, Bordia A, Verma SK. Curcumin, a major component of food spice turmeric (Curcuma longa) inhibits aggregation and alters eicosanoid metabolism in human blood platelets. *Prostaglandins Leukot Essent Fatty Acids* 1995;52:223–227.

6. Huang HC, Jan TR, Yeh SF. Inhibitory effect of curcumin, an anti-inflammatory agent, on vascular smooth muscle cell proliferation. *Eur J Pharmacol* 1992;221:381–384.

7. Ammon HP, Safayhi H, et al. Mechanism of anti-inflammatory actions of curcumine and boswellic acids. *J Enthopharmacol* 1993;38: 113–119.

8. Kulkarni RR, Patki PS, et al. Treatment of osteoarthritis with a herbomineral formulation: a double-blind, placebo-controlled, crossover study. *J Ethnopharmacol* 1991;33:91–95.

9. Mehta K, Pantazis P, et al. Antiproliferative effect of curcumin (diferuloylmethane) against human breast tumor cell lines. *Anticancer Drugs* 1997;8:470–481.

10. Hanif R, Qiao L, et al. Curcumin, a natural plant phenolic food additive, inhibits cell proliferation and induces cell cycle changes in colon adenocarcinoma cell lines by a prostaglandin-independent pathway. *J Lab Clin Med* 1997;130:576–584.

11. Goud VK, Olasa K, Krishnaswamy K. Effect of turmeric on xenobiotic metabolising enzymes. *Plant Foods Hum Nutr* 1993;44:87–92.

12. Aspisariyakul A, Vanittanakom N, Buddhasukh D. Antifungal activity of turmeric oil extracted from Curcuma longa (Zingiberaceae). *J Enthopharmacol* 1995;49:163–169.

13. Barthelemy S, Vergnes L, et al. Curcumin and curcumin derivatives inhibit Tat-mediated transactivation of type 1 human immunodeficiency virus long terminal repeat. *Res Virol* 1998;149:43–52.

ECHINACEA PURPUREA/ECHINACEA

1. Roesler J, Steinmuller C, et al. Application of purified polysaccharides from cell cultures of the plant Echinacea purpurea to mice mediates protection against systemic infections with Listeria monocytogenes and Candida albicans. *Int J Immunopharmacol* 1991;13:27–37.

2. Burger RA, Torres AR, et al. Echinacea-induced cytokine production by human macrophages. *Int J Immunopharmacol* 1997;19:371–379.

3. Wildfeuer A, Mayerhofer D. The effects of plant preparations on cellular functions in body defense. *Arzneimittelforschung* 1994;44:361–366.

4. Tubaro A, Tragni E, et al. Anti-inflammatory activity of a polysaccharide fraction of Echinacea augustifolia. *J Pharm Pharmacol* 1987;39:567–569.

5. Melchart D, Linde K, et al. Results of five randomized studies on the immunomodulatory activity of preparation of Echinacea. *J Altern Complement Med* 1995;1:145–160.

6. Elasser-Beile U, Willenbacher W, et al. Cytokine production in leukocyte cultures during therapy with Echinacea extract. *J Clin Lab Anal* 1996;10:441–445.

7. Melchart D, Linde K, et al. Immunomodulation with Echinacea: a systematic review of controlled clinical trials. *Phytomedicine* 1994;1:245–254.

8. Braunig B, Dorn M, et al. Echinacea purpurea Radix for strengthening the immune response in flu-like infections. *Z Phytother* 1992;13:7–13.

9. Schoeneberger D. The influence of immune-stimulating effects of pressed juice from Echinace purpurea on the course and severity of colds. *Forum Immunologie* 1992;8:2–12.

10. Melchart D, Walther E, et al. Echinacea root extracts for the prevention of upper respiratory tract infections: a double-blind, placebo-controlled randomized trial. *Arch Fam Med* 1998;7:541–545.

11. Grimm W, Muller HH. A randomized controlled trial of the effect of fluid extract of Echinacea purpurea on the incidence and severity of colds and respiratory infections. *Am J Med* 1999;106:138–143.

12. Brinkeborn RM, Shah DV, Degenring FH. Echinaforce and other Echinacea fresh plant preparations in the treatment of the common cold. A randomized, placebo-controlled, double-blind clinical trial. *Phytomedicine* 1999;6:1–5.

13. See DM, Broumand N, et al. In vitro effects of echinacea and ginseng on natural killer an antibody-dependent cell cytotoxicity in healthy subjects and chronic fatigue syndrome or acquired immunodeficiency syndrome patients. *Immunopharmacology* 1997;35:229–235.

14. Parnham MJ. Benefit-risk assessment of the squeezed sap of the purple coneflower (Echinacea purpurea) for long-term oral immunostimulation. *Phytomedicine* 1996;3:95–102.

15. Mengs U, Clare CB, Poiley JA. Toxicity of Echinacea purpurea. Acute, subacute, and genotoxicity studies. *Arzneimittelforschung* 1991;41:1076–1081.

16. Mullins RJ. Echinacea-associated anaphylaxis. *Med J Aust* 1998;168:170–171.

ELETTERIA CARDAMOMUM/CARDAMOM

1. al-Zuhair H, el-Sayeh B, et al. Pharmacological studies of cardamom oil in animals. *Pharmacol Res* 1996;34:79–82.

2. Huang YB, Hsu LR, et al. Crude drug (zingiberaceae) enhancement of percutaneous absorption of indomethacin: in vitro and in vivo permeation. *Kao Hsiung I Hsueh Ko Hsueh Tsa Chih* 1993;9:392–400.

3. Yamahara J, Kashiwa H, et al. Dermal penetration enhancement by crude drugs: in vitro skin permeation of prednisolone enhanced by active constituents in cardamom seed. *Chem Pharm Bull (Tokyo)* 1989;37:855–856.

4. Liu JQ, Wu DW. 32 cases of postoperative osteogenic sarcoma treated by chemotherapy combined with Chinese medicinal herbs. *Chung Kuo Chung Hsi I Chieh Ho Tsa Chih* 1993;13:50–52.

EMBLICA OFFICINALIS/AMALAKI

1. Kapoor LD. Emblica officinalis. In *Handbook of Ayurvedic Medicinal Plants,* 1990. CRC Press, Baca Raton, FL, p. 175.

2. Nandi P, Talukder G, Sharma A. Dietary chemoprevention of clastogenic effects of 3,4-benzo(a) pyrene by Emblica officinalis Gaertn. fruit extract. *Br J Cancer* 1997;76:1279–1283.

3. Grover IS, Kaur S. Effect of Emblica officinalis Gaertn. (Indian gooseberry) fruit extract on sodium azide and 4-nitro-phenylenediamine induced mutagenesis in Salmonella typhimurium. *Indian J Exp Biol* 1989;27:207–209.

4. Sharma HM, Dwivedi C, et al. Antineoplastic properties of Maharishi-4 (MAK-4) against DMBA-induced mammary tumors in rats. *Pharm Biochem Behav* 1990;35:767–773.

5. Patel VK, Wang J, et al. Reduction of metastases of Lewis lung carcinoma by an Ayurvedic food supplement (MAK-4) in mice. *Nutrition Res* 1992;12:51–61.

6. Thakur CP. Emblica officinalis reduces serum, aortic and hepatic cholesterol in rabbits. *Experientia* 1985;15:423–424.

7. Thakur CP, Thakur B, et al. The Ayurvedic medicines haritaki, amala and bahira reduce cholesterol-induced atherosclerosis in rabbits. *Int J Cardio* 1988;21:167–175.

8. Mathur R, Sharma A, et al. Hypolipidaemic effect of fruit juice of Emblica officinalis in cholesterol-fed rabbits. *J Ethnopharmacol* 1996;50:61–68.

9. Jacob A, Pandey M, et al. Effect of the Indian gooseberry (amla) on serum cholesterol levels in men aged 35–55 years. *Eur J Clin Nutr* 1988;42:939–944.

10. Sundaram V, Hanna AN, et al. The effect of oral herbal mixtures Maharishi Amrot Halask (MAK-4 and MAK-5) on lipoproteins and LDL oxidation in hyperlipidemic patients. *J Investig Med* 1995;43(Suppl. 3):483A (Abstract).

11. Sharma H, Feng Y, Panganamala RV. Maharishi Amrit Kalash (MAK-5) prevents human platelet aggregation. *Clinica and Terpia Cardiovascolare* 1989;8:227–230.

12. Chawla YK, Dubey P, et al. Treatment of dyspepsia with amalaki (Emblica officinalis Linn.)—an Ayurvedic drug. *Indian J Med Res* 1982;76(Suppl.):95–98.

13. Thorat SP, Rege NN, et al. Emblica officinalis: a novel therapy for acute pancreatitis—an experimental study. *HPB Surg* 1995;9:25–30.

14. Ahmad I, Mehmood Z, Mohammad F. Screening of some Indian medicinal plans for their antimicrobial properties. *J Ethnopharmacol* 1998;62:183–93.

GINGKO BILOBA/GINGKO

1. Auquet M, Delaflotte S, et al. The pharmacological basis for the vascular impact of Gingko Biloba extract. In *Rokan (Gingko biloba)—Recent Results in Pharmacology and Clinic.* Funfgeld EW (ed.) New York: Springer-Verlag, 1988;169–179.

2. Schaffler VK, Reeh PW. Double-blind study of the hypoxia-protective effect of a standardized Gingko bilobae preparation after repeated administration in healthy volunteers. *Arzneim-Forsch* 1985;35:1283–1286.

3. Karcher L, Zagerman P, Krieglstein J. Effect of an extract of Gingko biloba on rat brain energy metabolism in hypoxia. *Naunyn-Schmiedenberg's Arch Pharmacol* 1984;327:31–35.

4. Hofferberth B. Effect of Gingko biloba extract on neurophysiological and psychometric measurements in patients with cerebro-organic syndrome—a double-blind study versus placebo. *Arzneim Forsch* 1989;39:918–922.

5. Gessner B, Voelp A, Klasser M. Study of the long-term action of a Gingko biloba extract on vigilance and mental performance as determined by means of quantitative pharmaco-EEG and psychometric measurements. *Arzneim Forsch* 1985;35:1459–1465.

6. Maurer K, Ihl R, et al. Clinical efficacy of Gingko biloba special extract EGb 761 in dementia of the Alzheimer type. *J Psychiatr Res* 1997;31:645–655.

7. Kanowski S, Herrmann WM, et al. Proof of efficacy of the gingko biloba special extract EGb 761 in outpatients suffering from mild to moderate primary degenerative dementia of the Alzheimer type or multi-infarct dementia. *Pharmacopsychiatry* 1996;29:47–56.

8. Le Bars PL, Katz MM, et al. A placebo-controlled, double-blind, randomized trial of an extract of Gingko biloba for dementia. North American EGb study group. *JAMA* 1997;278:1327–1332.

9. Stoll S, Scheuer K, et al. Gingko biloba extract (EGb 761) independently improves changes in passive avoidance learning and brain membrane fluidity in the aging mouse. *Pharmacopsychiatry* 1996;29:144–149.

10. Cohen-Salmon C, Venault P, et al. Effects of Gingko biloba extract (EGb 761) on learning and possible actions on aging. *J Physiol Paris* 1997;91:291–300.

11. Wesnes KA, Faleni RA, et al. The cognitive, subjective, and physical effects of a gingko biloba/panax ginseng combination in healthy volunteers with neurasthenic complaints. *Psychopharmacol Bull* 1997;33:677–683.

12. Blume J, Kieser M, Holscher U. Placebo-controlled double-blind study of the effectiveness of Gingko biloba special extract EGb 761 in trained patients with intermittent claudication. *Vasa* 1996;25:265–274.

13. Letzel H, Schoop W. Gingko biloba extract Egb761 and pentoxifylline in intermittent claudication. Secondary analysis of the clinical effectiveness. *Vasa* 1992;21:403–410.

14. Drabaek H, Petersen JR, et al. The effect of Gingko biloba extract in patients with intermittent claudication. *Ugeskr Laeger* 1996;158:3928–3931.

15. Stange G, Benning CD, et al. Adaptational behaviour of peripheral and central acoustic responses in guinea pigs under the influence of various fractions of an extract from Gingko biloba. *Arzneimittelforschung* 1976;26:367–374.

16. Tighilet B, Lacour M. Pharmacological activity of the Gingko biloba extract (EGb 761) on equilibrium function recovery in the unilateral vestibular neurectomized cat. *J Vestib Res* 1995;5:187–200.

17. Cano Cuenco B, Marco Algarra J, et al. The effect of gingko biloba on cochleovestibulary pathology of vascular origin. *An Otorrinolaringol Ibero Am* 1995;22:619–629.

18. Roncin JP, Schwartz F, D'Arbigny P. EGb 761 in control of acute mountain sickness and vascular reactivity to cold exposure. *Aviat Space Environ Med* 1996;67:444–452.

19. Guinot P, Brambilla C, et al. Effect of BN 52063, a specific PAF-acether antagonist, on bronchial provocation test to allergens in asthmatic patients. A preliminary study. *Prostaglandins* 1987;34:723–31.

20. Cohen AJ, Bartlik B. Gingko biloba for anti-depressant-induced sexual dysfunction. *J Sex Marital Ther* 1998;24:139–143.

21. Sandberg-Gertzen H. An open trial of Cedemin, a Gingko biloba extract with PAF-antagonistic effects for ulcerative colitis. *Am J Gastroenterol* 1993;88:615–616.

22. Satyan KS, Jaiswal AK, et al. Anxiolytic activity of ginkgolic acid conjugates from Indian Gingko biloba. *Psychopharmacology (Berl)* 1998;136:148–152.

23. Tamborini A, Taurelle R. Value of standardized Gingko biloba extract (Egb 761) in the management of congestive symptoms of premenstrual syndrome. *Rev Fr Gynecol Obstet* 1993;88:447–457.

24. Turcan M, Cozmei C, et al. Effect of the EGb 761 (Gingko biloba) extract on primary immune response in experimental chronic stress. *Rev Med Chir Soc Med Nat Iasi* 1995;99:154–159.

25. Pietri S, Seguin JR, et al. Gingko biloba extract (EGb 761) in pretreatment limits free radical-induced oxidative stress in patients undergoing coronary bypass surgery. *Cardiovasc Drugs Ther* 11:121–131.

26. Koc Rk, Akdemir H, et al. Lipid peroxidation in experimental spinal cord injury. Comparison of treatment with Gingko biloba, TRH and methylprednisolone. *Res Exp Med (Berl)* 1995;195:117–123.

27. Rosenblatt M, Mindel J. Spontaneous hyphema associated with ingestion of Gingko biloba extract. *N Engl J Med* 1997;336:1108.

28. Rowin J, Lewis SL. Spontaneous bilateral subdural hematoma associated with Gingko biloba extract. *Neurology* 1996;46:1775–1776.

GLYCYRRHIZA GLABRA/LICORICE

1. Azimov MM, Zakirov UB, Radzhapova ShD. Pharmacological study of the anti-inflammatory agent glyderinine. *Farmakol Toksikol* 1988;51:90–93.

2. Vaya J, Belinky PA, Aviram M. Antioxidant constituents from licorice roots: isolation, structure elucidation and antioxidative capacity toward LDL oxidation. *Free Radic Biol Med* 1997;23:302–313.

3. Agarwal R, Wang ZY, Mukhtar H. Inhibition of mouse skin tumor-initiating activity of DMBA by chronic oral feeding of glycyrrhizin in drinking water. *Nutr Cancer* 1991;15:187–193.

4. Sitohy MZ, el-Massry RA, et al. Metabolic effects of licorice roots (Glycyrrhiza glabra) on lipid distribution pattern, liver and renal functions of albino rats. *Nahrung* 1991;35:799–806.

5. Francischetti IM, Monteiro RQ, Guimaraes JA. Identification of glycyrrhizin as a thrombin inhibitor. *Biochem Biophys Res Commun* 1997;237:203.

6. Moon A, Kim SH. Effect of Glycyrrhiza glabra roots and glycyrrhizin on the glucuronidation in rats. *Planta Med* 1997;63:115–119.

7. Pompei R, Flore O, et al. Glycyrrhizic acid inhibits virus growth and inactivates virus particles. *Nature* 1979;281:689–690.

8. Sato H, Goto W, et al. Therapeutic basis of glycyrrhizin on chronic hepatitis B. *Antiviral Res* 1996;30:171–177.

9. Shinada M, Azuma M, et al. Enhancement of interferon-gamma production in gylcyrrhizin-treated human peripheral lymphocytes in response to concanavalin A and to surface antigen of hepatitis B virus. *Proc Soc Exp Biol Med* 1986;181:205–210.

10. Nose M, Terawaki K, et al. Activation of macrophages by crude polysaccharide fractions obtained from shoots of Glycyrrhiza

glabra and hairy roots of Glycyrrhiza uralensis in vitro. *Biol Pharm Bull* 1998;21: 1110–1112.

11. Nadar TS, Pillai MM. Effect of ayurvedic medicines on beta-glucorinidase activity of Brunner's glands during recovery from cysteamine induced duodenal ulcers in rats. *Indian J Exp Biol* 1989;27:959–962.

12. Revers FE. Heeft succus liquiritiae een genezender werking op demaagzweer? *Ned Tÿdschr Geneeskd* 1946;90:135–137.

13. Basso A, Dalla Paola L, et al. Licorice ameliorates postural hypotension caused by diabetic autonomic neuropathy. *Diabetes Care* 1994;17:1356.

14. Baschetti R. Chronic fatigue syndrome and liquorice. *N Z Med J* 1995;108:156–157.

15. Stormer FC, Reistad R, J Alexander. Glycyrrhizic acid in liquorice—evaluation of health hazard. *Food Chem Toxicol* 1993;31: 303–312.

16. Bernardi M, D'Intino PE, et al. Effects of prolonged ingestion of graded doses of licorice by healthy volunteers. *Life Sci* 1994;55: 863–872.

Gymnema sylvestre/Gurmar

1. Arai K, Ishima R, et al. Three-dimensional structure of gurmarin, a sweet taste-suppressing polypeptide. *J Biomol NMR* 5: 297–305.

2. Shimizu K, Iino A, et al. Suppression of glucose absorption by some fractions extracted from Gymnema sylvestre leaves. *J Vet Med Sci* 1997;59:245–251.

3. Yoshikawa M, Murakami T, Matsuda H. Medicinal foodstuffs. X. Structure of new triterpene glycosides, gymnemosides-c, -e, -e, and -f, from the leaves of Gymnema sylvestre R. BR.: influence of gymnema glycosies on glucose uptake in rat small intestinal fragments. *Chem Phamr Bull (Tokyo)* 1997;45:2034–2038.

4. Wang LF, Luo H, et al. Inhibitory effect of gymnemic acid on intestinal absorption of oleic acid in rats. *Can J Physiol Pharmacol* 1998;76:1017–1023.

5. Shimizu K, Abe T, et al. Inhibitory effects of glucose utilization by gymnema acids in the guinea-pig ileal longitudinal muscle. *J Smooth Muscle Res* 1996;32:219–228.

6. Chattopadhyay RR. Possible mechanism of antihyperglycemic effect of Gymnema sylvestre leaf extract, part I. *Gen Pharmacol* 1998;31:495–496.

7. Nakamura Y, Tsumura Y, et al. Fecal steroid excretion is increased in rats by oral administration of gymnemic acids contained in Gymnema sylvestre leaves. *J Nutr* 1999;129: 1214–1222.

8. Shanmugasundaram ER, Gopinath KL, et al. Possible regeneration of the islets of Langerhans in streozotocin-diabetic rats given Gymnema sylvestres leaf extracts. *J Ethnopharmacol* 1990;30:265–279.

9. Shanmugasundaram ER, Rajeswari G, et al. Use of Gymnema sylvestre leaf extract in the control of blood glucose in insulin-dependent diabetes mellitus. *J Ethnopharmacol* 1990;30: 281–294.

10. Baskaran K, Kizar Ahamath B, et al. Antidiabetic effect of a leaf extract from Gymnema sylvestre in non-insulin-dependent diabetes mellitus patients. *J Ethnopharmacol* 1990;30: 295–300.

11. Min BC, Sakamoto K. Influence of sweet suppressing agent on gustatory brain evoked potentials generated by taste stimuli. *Appl Human Sci* 1998;17:9–17.

12. Brala PM, Hagen RL. Effects of sweetness perception and caloric value of a preload on short term intake. *Physiol Behav* 1983;30:1–9.

13. Gupta AA, Seth CB, Mathus VS. Effect of gurmar and shilajit on bodyweight of young rats. *Indian J Physiol Pharmacol* 1966;9:87–92.

1. Erdelmeier CA. Hyperforin, possibly the major non-nitrogenous secondary metabolite of Hypericum perforatum L. *Pharmacopsychiatry* 1998;31 Suppl 1:2–6.

2. Chatterjee SS, Noldner M, et al. Antidepressant activity of hypericum perforatum and hyperforin: the neglected possibility. *Pharmacopsychiatry* 1998;31 Suppl 1:7–15.

3. Muller WE, Singer A, et al. Hyperfroin represents the neurotransmitter reuptake inhibiting constituent of hypericum extract. *Pharmacopsychiatry* 1998;31 Suppl 1:16–21.

4. Chatterjee SS, Bhattacharya SK, et al. Hyperforin as a possible antidepressant component of hypericum extracts. *Life Sci* 1998;499:510.

5. Suzuki O, Katsumata Y, et al. Inhibition of monoamine oxidase by hypericin. *Planta Med* 1984;50:272–74.

6. Bladt S, Wagner H. Inhibition of MAO by fractions and constituents of hypericum extract. *J Geriatr Psychiatry Neurol* 1994;7 Suppl 1:S57–9.

7. Thiede HM, Walper A. Inhibition of MAO and COMT by hypericum extracts and hypericin. *J Geriatr Psychiatry Neurol* 1994;7 Suppl. 1:S54–6.

8. Baureithel KH, Buter KB, et al. Inhibition of benzodiazepine binding in vitro by amentoflavone, a constituent of various species of Hypericum. *Pharm Acta Helv* 1997;72:153–157.

9. Linde K, Ramirez G, et al. St. John's wort for depression—an overview and meta-analysis of randomised clinical trials. *BMJ* 1996;313:253–258.

10. Vorbach EU, Arnoldt KH, Hubner WD. Efficacy and tolerability of St. John's wort extract LI 160 versus imipramine in patients with severe depressive episodes according to ICD-10. *Pharmacopsychiatry* 1997;30 Suppl 2:81–85.

11. Wheatley D. LI 160, an extract of St. John's wort, versus amitriptyline in mildly to moderately depressed outpatients—a controlled 6-week clinical trial. *Pharmacopsychiatry* 1997;30 Suppl 2:77–80.

12. Nordfors M, Hartvig P. St. John's wort against depression in favour again. *Lakartidningen* 1997;94:2365–2367.

13. Schmidt U, Sommer H. St. John's wort extract in the ambulatory therapy of depression. *Fortschr Med* 1993;111:339–342.

14. Kasper S. Treatment of seasonal affective disorder (SAD) with hypericum extract. *Pharmacopsychiatry* 1997;30 Suppl 2:89–93.

15. Meruelo D, Lavie G, Lavie D. Therapeutic agents with dramatic antiretroviral activity and little toxicity at effective doses: aromatic polycyclic diones hypericin and pseudohypericin. *Proc Natl Acad Sci USA* 1988;85:5230–5234.

16. Takahashi I, Nakanishi S, et al. Hypericin and pseudohypericin specifically inhibit protein kinase C: possible relation to their antiretroviral activity. *Biochem Biophys Res Commun* 1989;165:1207–1212.

17. American Botanical Council. American Herbal Pharmacoepeia and Therapeutic Compendium. St. John's wort monograph. *HerbalGram* 1997;40:37–45.

18. Bol'shakova IV, Lozovskaia EL, Sapezhinskii II. Antioxidant properties of a series of extracts from medicinal plants. *Biofizika* 1997;42:480–483.

19. Bork PM, Bacher S, et al. Hypericin as a non-antioxidant inhibitor of NF-kappa B. *Planta Med* 1999 May;65(4):297–300.

20. Zhang W, Hinton DR, et al. Malignant glioma sensitivity to radiotherapy, high-dose tamoxifen, and hypericin: corroborating clinical response in vitro: case report. *Neurosurgery* 1996;38:587–590.

21. Zhang W, Anker L, et al. Enhancement of radiosensitivity in human malignant glioma cells by hypericin in vitro. *Clin Cancer Res* 1996;2:843–846.

22. Miller AL. St. John's wort (Hypericum perforatum): clinical effects on depression and other conditions. *Altern Med Rev* 1998;3: 18–26.

23. Monmaney T. St. John's wort: Regulatory vacuum leaves doubt about potency, effects of herb used for depression. *Los Angeles Times,* August 31, 1998, front page.

24. Golsch S, Vocks E, et al. Reversible increase in photosensitivity to UV-B caused by St. John's wort extract. *Hautarzt* 1997;48:249–252.

LAVENDULA ANGUSTIFOLIA/LAVENDER

1. Wan J, Wolcock A. Coventry MJ. The effect of essential oils of basil on the growth of Aeromonas hydrophilia and Pseudomonas flourescens. *J Appl Microbiol* 1998;84:152–158.

2. Inouye S, Watanabe M, et al. Antisporulating and respiration-inhibitory effects of essential oils on filamentous fungi. *Mycoses* 1998;41: 403–410.

3. Cornwell S, Dale A. Lavender oil and perineal repair. *Mod Midwife* 1995;5:31–33.

4. Buchbauer G, Jirovetz L, et al. Fragrance compounds and essential oils with sedative effects upon inhalation. *J Pharm Sci* 1993;82:660–664.

5. Dleaveay P, Guillemain J, et al. Neurodepressive properties of essential oil of lavender. *C R Seances Soc Biol Fil* 1989;183: 342–348.

6. Bradshaw RH, Marchant JN, et al. Effects of lavender straw on stress and travel sickness in pigs. *J Altern Complement Med* 1998;4:271–275.

7. Alaoui-Ismaili O, Vernet-Maury E, et al. Odor hedonics: connection with emotional response estimated by autonomic parameters. *Chem Senses* 1997;22:237–248.

8. Dunn C, Sleep J, Collett D. Sensing an improvement: an experimental study to evaluate the use of aromatherapy, massage and periods of rest in an intensive care unit. *J Adv Nurs* 1995;21:34–40.

9. Hay IC, Jamieson M, Ormerod AD. Randomized trial of aromatherapy. Successful treatment for alopecia areata. *Arch Dermatol* 1998;134:1349–1352.

LINUM USITATISSIMUM/FLAXSEED

1. Prasad K, Mantha SV, et al. Reduction of hypercholesterolemic atherosclerosis by CDC-flaxseed with very low alpha-linolenic acid. *Atherosclerosis* 1998;136:357–375.

2. Prasad K. Reduction of serum cholesterol and hypercholesterolemic atherosclerosis in rabbits by secoisolariciresinol diglucoside isolated from flaxseed. *Circulation* 1999;99: 1355–1362.

3. Jenkins DJ, Kendall CW, et al. Health aspects of partially defatted flaxseed, including effects on serum lipids, oxidative measures, and ex vivo androgen and progestin activity: a controlled crossover trial. *Am J Clin Nutr* 1999;69:395–402.

4. Cunnane SC, Hamadeh MJ, et al. Nutritional attributes of traditional flaxseed in healthy young adults. *Am J Clin Nutr* 1995;61:62–68.

5. Thompson LU, Rickard SE, et al. Flaxseed and its lignan and oil components reduce mammary tumor growth at a late stage of carcinogenesis. *Carcinogenesis* 1996;17:1373–1376.

6. Sung MK, Lautens M, Thompson LU. Mammalian lignans inhibit the growth of estrogen-independent human colon tumor cells. *Anticancer Res* 1998;18(3A):1405–1408.

7. Yan L, Yee JA, et al. Dietary flaxseed supplementation and experimental metastasis of melanoma cells in mice. *Cancer Lett* 1998;127: 181–186.

8. Haggans CJ, Hutchins AM, et al. Effect of flaxseed consumption on urinary estrogen metabolites in postmenopausal women. *Nutr Cancer* 1999;33:188–195.

9. Kurzer MS, Lampe JW, et al. Fecal lignan and isoflavonoid excretion in premenopausal women consuming flaxseed powder. *Cancer Epidemiol Biomarkers Prev* 1995;4:353–358.

10. Nordstrom DC, Honkanen VE, et al. Alpha-linolenic acid in the treatment of rheumaoid arthritis. A double-blind, placebo-controlled and randomized study: flaxseed vs. safflower seed. *Rheumatol Int* 1995;14:231–234.

11. Clark WF, Parbtani A, et al. Flaxseed: a potential treatment for lupus nephritis. *Kidney Int* 1995;48:475–480.

12. See note 4 above.

MELALEUCA ALTERNIFOLIA/TEA TREE

1. Williams LR. Clonal production of tea tree oil high in terpinen-4-ol for use in formulations for the treatment of thrush. *Complement Ther Nurs Midwifery* 1998;4:133–136.

2. Tong MM, Altman PM, Barnetson RS. Tea tree oil in the treatment of tinea pedis. *Australas J Dermatol* 1992;33:145–149.

3. Buck DS, Nidorf DM, Addino JG. Comparison of two topical preparations for the treatment of onychomycosis: Melaleuca alternifolia (tea tree) oil and clotrimazole. *J Fam Pract* 1994;38:601–605.

4. Nenoff P, Haustein UF, Brandt W. Antifungal activity of the essential oil of Melaleuca alternifolia (tea tree oil) against pathogenic fungi in vitro. *Skin Pharmacol* 1996;9:388–394.

5. Hammer KA, Carson CF, Riley TV. In-vitro activity of essential oils, in particular Melaleuca alternifolia (tea tree oil) and tea tree oil products, against Candida spp. *J Antimicrob Chemother* 1998;42:591–595.

6. Hammer KA, Carson CF, Riley TV. Susceptibility of transient and commensual skin flora to the essential oil of Melaleuca alternifolia (tea tree oil). *Am J Infect Control* 1996;24:186–189.

7. Raman A, Weir U, Bloomfield SF. Antimicrobial effects of tea-tree oil and its major components on Staphyloccus aureus, Staph. Epidermidis and Propionibacterium acnes. *Lett Appl Microbiol* 1995;21:242–245.

8. Bassett AB, Pannowitz DL, Barnetson RS. A comparative study of tea-tree oil versus benzoylperoxide in the treatment of acne. *Med J Aust* 1990;153:455–458.

9. Faoagali J, George N, Leditschke JF. Does tea tree oil have a place in the topical treatment of burns? *Burns* 1997;23:349–351.

10. Carson CF, Cookson BD, et al. Susceptibility of methicillin-resistant Staphlococcus aureus to the essential oil of Melaleuca alternifolia. *J Antimicrob Chemother* 1995;35:421–424.

11. Pena EF. Melaleuca alternifolia oil. *Obstet Gynecol* 1962;19:793–795.

12. Wolner-Hanssen P, Sjoberg I. Warning against a fashionable cure for vulvovaginitis. Tea tree oil may substitute Candida itching with allergy itching. *Lakartidningen* 1998;95:3309–3310.

13. Rubel DM, Freeman S, Southwell IA. Tea tree oil allergy: what is the offending agent? Report of three cases of tea tree oil allergy and review of the literature. *Australas J Dermatol* 1998;39:244–247.

14. Knight TE, Hausen BM. Melaleuca oil (tea tree) dermatitis. *J Am Acad Dermatol* 1994;30:423–427.

15. Jacobs MR, Hornfeldt CS. Melaleuca oil poisoning. *J Toxicol Clin Toxicol* 1994;32:461–464.

MUCUNA PRURIENS/ATMAGUPTA

1. Rajyalakshmi P, Geervani P. Nutritive value of the foods cultivated and consumed by the tribals of south India. *Plant Foods Hum Nutr* 1994;46:53–61.

2. Vijayakumari K, Siddhuraju P, Janardhanan K. Effect of different post-harvest treatments

on antinutritional factors in seeds of the tribal pulse, Mucina pruriens (L.) DC. *Int J Food Sci Nutr* 1996;47:263–272.

3. Manyam BV. Paralysis agitans and levodopa in "Ayurveda": ancient Indian medical treatise. *Mov Disord* 1990;5:47–48.

4. Pras N, Woerdenbag HJ, et al. Mucuna pruriens: improvement of the biotechnological production of the anti-Parkinson drug L-dopa by plant cell selection. *Pharm World Sci* 1993;15:263–268.

5. An alternative medicine treatment for Parkinson's disease: results of a multicenter clinical trial. HP-200 in Parkinson's Disease Study Group. *J Altern Complement Med* 1995;1: 249–255.

6. Vaidya AB, Rajagopalan TG, et al. Treatment of Parkinson's disease with the cowhage plant— Mucuna pruriens. *Neurology India* 26:171–176.

7. Akhtar MS, Qureshi AQ, Iqbal J. Antidiabetic evaluation of Mucuna pruriens, Linn seeds. *J Pak Med Assoc* 1990;40:147–150.

8. Pant MC, Uddin I, et al. Blood sugar and total cholesterol lowering effect of gylcine soja (Sieb and Zucc.), Mucuna pruriens (D.C.) and Dolichos biflous (Linn.) seed diets in normal and fasting albino rats. *Ind J Med Res* 1968;56:1808–1812.

9. Hoghton PJ, Skari KP. The effect on blood clotting of some west African plants used against snakebite. *J Ethnopharmacol* 1994;44:99–108.

10. No author listed. Mucuna pruriens–associated pruritis—New Jersey. *JAMA* 1986;255:313.

11. Infante ME, Perez AM, et al. Outbreak of acute toxic psychosis attributed to Mucuna pruriens. *Lancet* 1990;336:1129.

OCIMUM SANCTUM/TULSI

1. Maulik G, Maulik N, et al. Evaluation of antioxidant effectiveness of a few herbal plants. *Free Radic Res* 1997;27:221–228.

2. Singh S, Majumdar DK. Evaluation of anti-inflammatory activity of fatty acids of Ocimum sanctum fixed oil. *Indian J Exp Biol* 1997;35:380–383.

3. Godhwani, S Godhwani JL, Vyas DS. Ocimum sanctum: an experimental study evaluating its anti-inflammatory, analgesic and antipyretic activity in animals. *J Ethnopharmacol* 1987;21:153–163.

4. Sen P, Maiti PC, et al. Mechanism of anti-stress activity of Ocimum sanctum Linn, eugenol and Tinospora malabarica in experimental animals. *Indian J Exp Biol* 1992;30:592–596.

5. Sakina MR, Dandiya PC, et al. Preliminary psychopharmacological evaluation of Ocimum sanctum leaf extract. *J Ethnopharmacol* 1990;28:143–150.

6. Sembulingam K, Sembulingam P, Namasivayam A. Effect of Ocimum sanctum Linn on noise induced changes in plasma corticosterone level. *Indian J Physiol Pharmacol* 1997;41:139–143.

7. Ganasoundari A, Devi PU, Rao BS. Enhancement of bone marrow radioprotection and reduction of WR-2721 toxicity by Ocimum sanctum. *Mutat Res* 1998;397:303–312.

8. Uma Devi P, Ganasoundari A, et al. In vivo radioprotection by ocimum flavonoids: survival of mice. *Radiat Res* 1999;151:74–78.

9. Devi PU, Bisht KS, Vinitha M. A comparative study of radioprotection by Ocimum flavonoids and synthetic aminothiol protectors in the mouse. *Br J Radiol* 1998;71: 782–784.

10. Balanehru S, Nagarajan B. Intervention of adriamycin induced free radical damage. *Biochem Int* 1992;28:735–744.

11. Karthikeyan K, Ravichandran P, Govindasamy S. Chemoprotective effect of Ocimum sanctum on DMBA-induced hamster buccal pouch carcinogenesis. *Oral Oncol* 1999;35:112–119.

12. Prashar R, Kumar A, et al. Inhibition by an extract of Ocimum sanctum of DNA-binding activity of 7,12-dimethylbenz[a]anthracene in hepatocytes in vitro. *Cancer Lett* 1998;128:155–160.

13. Godhwani S, Godhwani JL, Vyas DS. Ocimum sanctum—a preliminary study evaluating its immunoregulatory profile in albino rats. *J Ethnopharmacol* 1988;24:193–198.

14. Chattopadhyay RR. Hypoglycemic effect of Ocimum sanctum leaf extract in normal and streptozotocin diabetic rats. *Indian J Exp Biol* 1993;31:891–893.

15. Rai V, Iyer U, Mani UV. Effect of Tulasi (Ocimum sanctum) leaf powder supplementation on blood sugar levels, serum lipids and tissue lipids in diabetic rats. *Plant Foods Hum Nutr* 1997;50:9–16.

16. Sarkar A, Lavania SC, et al. Changes in the blood lipid profile after administration of Ocimum sanctum (Tulsi) leaves in the normal albino rabbits. *Indian J Physiol Pharmacol* 1994;38:311–312.

17. Agrawal P, Rai V, Singh RB. Randomized placebo-controlled, single blind trial of holy basil leaves in patients with noninsulin-dependent diabetes mellitus. *Int J Clin Pharmacol Ther* 1996;34:406–409.

18. Singh S, Majumdar DK. Evaluation of the gastric antiulcer activity of fixed oil of Ocimum sanctum. *J Ethnopharmacology* 1999;65:13–19.

19. Manda S, Das DN, et al. Ocimum sanctum Linn—a study on gastric ulceration and gastric secretion in rats. *Indian J Phyisol Pharmacol* 1993;37:91–92.

PHYLLANTHUS NIRURI/PHYLLANTHUS

1. Venkateswaran PS, Millman I, Blumberg BS. Effects of an extract from Phyllanthus niruri on hepatitis B and woodchuck hepatitis viruses: in vitro an din vivo studies. *Proc Nat Acad Sci USA* 1987;84:274–278.

2. Thyagarajan SP, Subramanian S, et al. Effects of Phyllanthus amarus on chronic carriers of hepatitis B virus. *Lancet* 1988 Oct 1;2:764–766.

3. Lee CD, Ott M, et al. Phyllanthus amarus down-regulates hepatitis B virus mRNA transcription and replication. *Eur J Clin Invest* 1996;26:1069–1076.

4. Yeh SF, Hong CY, et al. Effect of an extract from Phyllanthus amarus on hepatitis B surface antigen gene expression in human hepatoma cells. *Antiviral Res* 1993;20:185–192.

5. Thamlikitkul V, Wasuwat S, Kanchanepee P. Efficacy of Phyllanthus amarus for eradication of hepatitis B virus in chronic carriers. *J Med Assoc Thai* 1991;74:381–385.

6. Doshi JC, Vaidya AB, et al. A two-step clinical trial of Phyllanthus amarus in hepatitis B carriers: failure to eradicate the surface antigen. *Indian J Gastroenterol* 1994;13:7–8.

7. Liu KC, Lin MT, et al. Antiviral tannins from two Phyllanthus species. *Planta Med* 1999;65:43–46.

8. Ogata T, Higuchi H, et al. HIV-1 reverse transcriptase inhibitor from Phyllanthus niruri. *AIDS Res Hum Retroviruses* 1992;8:1937–1944.

9. Sebastian T, Setty OH. Protective effect of P. fraternus against ethanol-induced mitochondrial dysfunction. *Alcohol* 1999;17:29–34.

10. Syamasundar KV, Singh B, et al. Antihepatotoxic principles of Phyllanthus niruri herbs. *J Ethnopharmacol* 1985;14:41–44.

11. Calixto JB, Yunes RA, et al. Antispasmodic effects of an alkaloid extracted from Phyllanthus sellowianus: a comparative study with papaverine. *Braz J Med Biol Res* 1984;17:313–321.

12. Campos AH, Schor N. Phyllanthus niruri inhibits calcium oxalate endocytosis by renal tubular cells: its role in urolithiasis. *Nephron* 1999;81:393–397.

13. Srividya N, Periwal S. Diuretic, hypotensive and hypoglycaemic effect of Phyllanthus amarus. *Indian J Exp Biol* 1995;33:861–864.

14. Santos AR, Filho VC, et al. Analysis of the mechanisms underlying the antinociceptive effect of the extracts of plants from the genus Phyllanthus. *Gen Pharmacol* 1995;26: 1499–1506.

15. Ihantoala-Vormisto A, Summanen J, et al. Anti-inflammatory activity of extracts from the leaves of Phyllanthus emblica. *Planta Med* 1997;63:518–524.

PICRORHIZA KURROA/KUTKI

1. Chaturvedi GN, Singh RH. Treatment of jaundice with an indigenous drug *Picrorhiza kurroa*—a clinical and experimental study. *Curr Med Pract* 1965;9:451–453.

2. Dwivedi Y, Rastogi R, et al. Effects of picroliv, the active principle of Picrorhiza kurroa, on biochemical changes in rat liver poisoned by Amanita phalliodes. *Chung Kuo Yao Li Hsueh Pao* 1992;13:197–200.

3. Dwivedi Y, Rastogi R, et al. Perfusion with picroliv reverses biochemical changes induced in livers of rats toxicated with galactosamine or thioacetamide. *Planta Med* 1993;59: 418–420.

4. Vaidya AB, Antarkar DS, et al. Picrorhiza kurroa (Kutaki) Royle ex Benth as a hepato-protective agent—experimental & clinical studies. *J Postgrad Med* 1996;42:105–108.

5. Floersheim GL, Bieri A, et al. Protection against Amanita phalloides by the iridoid glycoside mixture of Picrorhiza kurroa (kutkin). *Agents Actions* 1990;29:386–387.

6. Mittal N, Gupta N, et al. Protective effect of picroliv from Picrorhiza kurroa against Leishmania donovani in Mesocricetus. *Life Sci* 1998;63:1823–1834.

7. Sinha M, Mehrotra J, et al. Picroliv, the iridoid glycoside fraction of Picrorhiza kurroa, selectively augments human T cell response to my-cobacterial protein antigens. *Immunopharmacol Immunotoxicol* 1998;30:579–588.

8. Rastogi R, Saksena S, et al. Picroliv protects against alcohol-induced chronic hepatotoxicity in rats. *Planta Med* 1996;62:283–285.

9. Mehrotra R, Rawat S, et al. In vitro studies on the effect of certain natural products against hepatitis B virus. *Indian J Med Res* 1990;92:133–138.

10. Shukla B, Visen PK, et al. Choleretic effect of picroliv, the hepatoprotective principle of Picrorhiza kurroa. *Planta Med* 1991;57: 29–33.

11. Luper S. A review of plants used in the treatment of liver disease: part 1. *Altern Med Rev* 1998;3:410–321.

12. Baruah CC, Gupta PP, et al. Anti-allergic and anti-anaphylactic activity of picroliv—a standardized iridoid glycoside fraction of Picrorhiza kurroa. *Pharmacol Res* 1998;38: 487–492.

13. Dorsch W, Stuooner H, et al. Antiasthmatic effects of Picrorhiza kurroa: androsin prevents allergin and PAF-induced bronchial obstruction in guinea pigs. *Int Arch Allergy Appl Immunol* 1991;95:128–133.

14. Engels F, Renirie BF, et al. Effects of apocynin, a drug isolated from the roots of Picrorhiza kurroa, on arachidonic acid metabolism. *FEBS Lett* 1992;305:254–256.

15. Dorsch W, Wagner H. New antiasthmatic drugs from traditional medicine? *Int Arch Allergy Appl Immunol* 1991;94:262–265.

16. Sharma ML, Rao CS, et al. Immunostimulatory activity of Picrorhiza kurroa leaf extract. *J Ethnopharmacol* 1994;41:185–192.

PIPER METHYSTICUM/KAVA KAVA

1. Kinzler E, Kromer J, Lehmann E. Effect of a special kava extract in patients with anxiety-, tension-, and excitation states of nonpsychotic genesis. Double blind study with placebos over 4 weeks. *Arzneimittelforschung* 1991;41: 585–588.

2. Volz HP, Kieser M. Kava-kava extract WS 1490 versus placebo in anxiety disorders—a randomized placebo-controlled 25-week outpatient trial. *Pharmacopsychiatry* 1997;30:1–5.

3. Scherer J. Kava-kava extract in anxiety disorders: an outpatient observational study. *Adv Ther* 1998;15:261–269.

4. Warnecke G. Psychosomatic dysfunctions in the female climacteric. Clinical effectiveness and tolerance of kava extract WS 1490. *Fortschr Med* 1991;119–122.

5. Munte TF, Heinze HJ, et al. Effects of oxazepam and an extract of kava roots (Piper methysticum) on event-related potentials in a word recognition task. *Neuropsychology* 1993; 27:46–53.

6. Heinze HJ, Munthe TF, et al. Pharmacopsychological effects of oxazepam and kava-extract in a visual search paradigm assessed with event-related potentials. *Pharmacopsychiatry* 1994;27:224–230.

7. Herberg KW. Effect of kava-special extract WS 1490 combined with ethyl alcohol on safety-relevant performance parameters. *Blutalkohol* 1993;30:96–105.

8. Langosch JM, Normann C, et al. The influence of (+/−) kavain on population spikes and long-term potentiation in guinea pig hippocampal slices. *Comp Biochem Physiol A Mol Integr Physiol* 1998;120:545–549.

9. Boonen G, Haberlein H. Influence of genuine kavapyrone enantiomers on the GABA-A binding site. *Planta Med* 1998;64:504–506.

10. Schmitz D, Zhang CL, et al. Effects of methysticin on three different models of seizure like events studied in rat hippocampal and entorhinal cortex slices. *Naunyn Schmiedebergs Arch Pharmacol* 1995;351:348–355.

11. Jamieson DD, Duffield PH. The antinociceptive actions of kava components in mice. *Clin Exp Pharmacol Physiol* 1990;17:495–507.

12. Backhauss C, Krieglstein J. Extract of kava (Piper methysticum) and its methysticin constituents protect brain tissue against ischemic damage in rodents. *Eur J Pharmacol* 1993;215: 265–269.

13. Duffield PH, Jamieson D. Development of tolerance to kava in mice. *Clin Exp Pharmacol Physiol* 1991;18:571–578.

14. Almeida JC, Grimsley EW. Coma from the health food store: interaction between kava and alprazolam. *Ann Intern Med* 1996;125: 940–941.

15. Strahl S, Ehret V, et al. Necrotizing hepatitis after taking herbal remedies. *Dtsch Med Wochenschr* 1998;123:1410–1414.

16. Norton SA, Ruze P. Kava dermopathy. *J Am Acad Dermatol* 1994;31:89–97.

17. Ruze P. Kava-induced dermopathy: a niacin deficiency? *Lancet* 1990;335:1442–1445.

18. Jappe U, Franke I, et al. Sebotropic drug reaction resulting from kava-kava extract therapy: a new entity? *J Am Acad Dermatol* 1998;38: 104–106.

19. Suss R, Lehmann P. Hematogenous contact eczema cause by phytogenic drugs exemplified by kava root extract. *Hautarzt* 1996;47:459–461.

SERENOA REPENS/SAW PALMETTO

1. Sultan C, Terraza A, et al. Inhibition of androgen metabolism and binding by a liposterolic extract of Serenoa repens B in human foreskin fibroblasts. *J Steroid Biochem* 1984;20:414–419.

2. Weisser H, Tunn S, et al. Effects of the sabal serrulata extract IDS 89 and its subfractions on 5 alpha-reductase activity in human benign prostatic hyperplasia. *Prostate* 1996;28:300–306.

3. Weisser H, Behnke B, et al. Enzyme activities in tissue of human benign prostatic hyperplasia after three months' treatment with Sabal serrulata extract IDS 89 (Strogen) or placebo. *Eur Urol* 1997;31:97–101.

4. Gutierrez M, Garcia de Boto MJ, et al. Mechanisms involved in the spasmolytic effect of extracts from Sabal serrulata fruit on smooth muscle. *Gen Pharmacol* 1996;27:171–176.

5. Goepel M, Hecker U, et al. Saw palmetto extracts potently and noncompetitively inhibit human alpha 1-adrenoceptors in vitro. *Prostate* 1999;38:210–215.

6. Breu W, Hagenlocher M, et al. Anti-inflammatory activity of sabal fruit extracts prepared with supercritical carbon dioxide. In vitro antagonists of cyclooxygenase and 5-lipoxygenase metabolism. *Arzneimittelforschung* 1992;42:547–551.

7. Carbin BE, Larsson B, Lindahl O. Treatment of benign prostatic hyperplasia with phytosterols. *Br J Urol* 1990;66:639–641.

8. Romics I, Schmits H, Frang D. Experience in treating benign prostatic hypertrophy with Sabal serrulata for one year. *Int Urol Nephrol* 1993;25:565–569.

9. Vahlensieck W, Volp A, et al. Benign prostatic hyperplasia—treatment with sabal fruit extract. A treatment of 1,334 patients. *Fortschr Med* 1993;111:323–326.

10. Kondas J, Phillips V, Dioszeghy G. Sabal serrulata extract (Strogen forte) in the treatment of symptomatic benign prostatic hyperplasia. *Int Urol Nephrol* 1996;28:767–772.

11. Gerber GS, Zagaja GP, et al. Saw palmetto (Serenoa repens) in men with lower urinary tract symptoms: effects on urodynamic parameters and voiding symptoms. *Urology* 1998; 51:1003–1007.

12. Wilt TJ, Ishana A, et al. Saw palmetto extract for treatment of benign prostatic hyperplasia: a systematic review. *JAMA* 1998;280:1604–1609.

13. Ondrizek RR, Chan PJ, et al. Inhibition of human sperm motility by specific herbs used in alternative medicine. *J Assist Reprod Genet* 1999;16:87–91.

SILYBUM MARIANUM/MILK THISTLE

1. Flora K, Hahn M, et al. Milk thistle (Silybum marianum) for the therapy of liver disease. *Am J Gastroenterol* 1998;93:139–143.

2. Schoepen RD, Lange OK, et al. Searching for a new therapeutic principle. Experience with hepatic therapeutic agent legalon. *Med Welt* 1969;20:888–893.

3. Schoepen RD, Lange OK. Therapy of hepatoses. Therapeutic use of silymarin. *Med Welt* 1970;21:691–698.

4. Magliulo E, Gagliardi B, Fiori GP. Zur Wirkung von Silymarin beider Behandlung der akuten Virushepatitis. *Med Klin* 1978;73.

5. Ferenci P, Dragosics B, et al. Randomized controlled trial of silymarin treatment in patients with cirrhosis of the liver. *J Hepatol* 1989;9:105–113.

6. Vogel G. Natural substances with effects on the liver. In *New Natural Products and Plant Drugs with Pharmacological, Biological or Therapeutical Activity.* New York: Springer-Verlag 1977:2651–2665.

7. Hikino H, Kiso Y, et al. Antihepatotoxic actions of flavanolignans from Silybum marianum fruits. *Planta Med* 1984;50: 248–250.

8. Kreeman V, Skottova N, et al. Silymarin inhibits the development of diet-induced hypercholesterolemia in rats. *Planta Med* 1998;64: 138–142.

9. Skottova N, Kreeman V. Silymarin as a potential hypocholesterolaemic drug. *Physiol Res* 1998;47:1–7.

10. Rui YC. Advances in pharmacological studies of silymarin. *Mem Inst Oswaldo Cruz* 1991;86 (Suppl 2):79–85.

TANACETUM PARTHENIUM/FEVERFEW

1. Makheja Am, Bailey JM. A platelet phosphlipase inhibitor from the medicinal herb fever-

few (Tanacetum parthenium). *Prostagland Leukotriene Med* 1982;8:653–660.

2. Pugh WJ, Sambo K. Prostaglandin synthetase inhibitors in feverfew. *J Pharm Pharmacol* 1988;40:743–745.

3. Hwang D, Fischer NH, et al. Inhibition of the expression of inducible cyclooxygenase and proinflammatory cytokines by sesquiterpene lactones in macrophages correlates with the inhibition of MAP kinases. *Biochem Biophys Res Commun* 1996;226:810–818.

4. Groenewegen WA, Heptinstall S. A comparison of the effects of an extract of feverfew and parthenolide, a component of feverfew, on human platelet activity in-vitro. *J Pharm Pharmacol* 1990;42:553–557.

5. Murch SJM, Simmons CB, Saxena PK. Melatonin in feverfew and other medicinal plants. *Lancet* 1997;350:1598–1599.

6. Vogler BK, Pittler MH, Ernst E. Feverfew as a preventive treatment for migraine: a systematic review. *Cephalalgia* 1998;18:704–708.

7. Johnson ES, Kadam NP, et al. Efficacy of feverfew as prophylactic treatment of migraine. *Br Med J* 1985;291:569–573.

8. Murphy JJ, Heptinstall S, Mitchell JR. Randomised double-blind placebo-controlled trial of feverfew in migraine prevention. *Lancet* 1988;ii:189–192.

9. Palevitch D, Earon G, Carasso R. Feverfew (Tanacetum parthenium) as a prophylactic treatment for migraine: a double-blind placebo-controlled study. *Phytother Res* 1997;11:508–511.

10. See note 7 above.

11. See note 8 above.

12. Pattrick M, Heptinstall S, Doherty M. Feverfew in rheumatoid arthritis: a double blind, placebo-controlled study. *Ann Rheum Dis* 1989;48:547–549.

13. Heptinstall S, Awang DVC, et al. Pathenolide content and bioactivity of feverfew (Tanacetum parthenium (L.) Schultz-Bip.). Estimation of commercial and authenticated feverfew products. *J Phamr Pharmacol* 1992;44:391–395.

TERMINALIA ARJUNA/ARJUNA

1. Patnaik N. Arjuna. In *The Garden of Life*. 1993. Doubleday, New York: p. 79.

2. Sahila HP, Udupa SI, Udupa AL. Hypolipidemic activity of three indigenous drugs in experimentally induced atherosclerosis. *Int J Cardiol* 1998;67:119–124.

3. Ram A, Lauria P, et al. Hypocholesterolaemic effects of Terminalia arjuna tree bark. *J Ethnopharmacol* 1997;55:165–169.

4. Dwivedi S, Agarwal MP. Antianginal and cardioprotective effects of Terminalia arjuna, an indigenous drug, in coronary artery disease. *J Assoc Physicians India* 1994;42:287–289.

5. Dwivedi S, Jauhari R. Beneficial effects of Terminalia arjuna in coronary artery disease. *Indian Heart J* 1997;49:507–510.

6. Bharani A, Ganguly A, Bhargava KD. Slautary effect of Terminallia arjuna in patients with severe refractory heart failure. *Int J Cardiol* 1995;49:191–199.

7. Seth SD, Maulik M, et al. Role of Lipistat in protection against isoproterenol induced myocardial necrosis in rats: a biochemical and histopathological study. *Indian J Phyisol Pharmacol* 1998;42:101–106.

8. Pettit GR, Hoard MS, et al. Antineoplastic agents 338. The cancer cell growth inhibitory constituents of Terminalia arjuna (Combretaceae). *J Ethnopharmacol* 1996;53:57–63.

9. Perumal Samy R, Ignacimuthu S, Sen A. Screening of 34 Indian medicinal plants for antibacterial properties. *J Ethnopharmacol* 1998;62:173–182.

TINOSPORA CORDIFOLIA/AMRIT

1. Kapil A, Sharma S. Immunopotentiating compounds from Tinospora cordifolia. *J Ethnopharmacol* 1997;58:89–95.
2. Dhuley JN. Effect of some Indian herbs on macrophage functions in ochratoxin A treated mice. *J Ethnopharmacol* 1997;58:15–20.
3. Thatte UM, Kulkarni MR, Dahanukar SA. Immunotherapeutic modification of Escherichia coli perotonitis and bacteremia by Tinospora cordifolia. *J Postgrad Med* 1992;38:13–15.
4. Rege NN, Dahanukar SA. Quantitation of microbicidal activity of mononuclear phago-cytes: an in vitro technique. *J Postgrad Med* 1993;39:22–25.
5. Sohni YR, Bhatt RM. Activity of a crude extract formulation in experimental hepatic amoebiasis and in immunomodulation studies. *J Ethnopharmacol* 1996;54:119–124.
6. Rege NN, Nazareth HM, et al. Modulation of immunosuppression in obstuctive jaundice by Tinospora cordifolia. *Indian J Med Res* 1989;90:478–483.
7. Bapat RD, Rege NN, et al. Can we do away with PTBD? *HPB Surg* 1995;9:5–11.
8. Rege N, Bapat RD, et al. Immunotherapy with Tinospora cordifolia: a new lead in the management of obstructive jaundice. *Indian J Gastroenterol* 1993;12:5–8.
9. Jagetia GC, Nayak V, Vidyasagar MS. Evaluation of the antineoplastic activity of guduchi (Tinospora cordifolia) in cultured HeLa cells. *Cancer Lett* 1998;127:71–82.
10. Mathew S, Kuttan G. Antioxidant activity of Tinospora cordifolia and its usefulness in the amelioration of cyclophosphamide induced toxicity. *J Exp Clin Cancer Res* 1997;16:407–411.
11. Wadood N, Wadood A, Shah SA. Effect of Tinospora cordifolia on blood glucose and total lipid levels of normal and alloxan-diabetic rabbits. *Planta Med* 1992;58:131–136.
12. Stanely Mainsen Prince P, Menon VP, Gu-nasekaran G. Hypolipidaemic action of Tinospora cordifolia roots in alloxan diabetic rats. *J Ethnopharmacol* 1999;63:53–57.
13. Rege NN, Thatte UM, Dahanukar SA. Adaptogenic properties of six rasayana herbs used in Ayurvedic medicine. *Phytother Res* 1999;13:275–291.

TRIGONELLA FOENUM-GRAECUM/FENUGREEK

1. Mowrey DB. Cholesterol regulation. In *The Scientific Validation of Herbal Medicine*. 1986, Keats Publishing, New Canaan, CT, p. 41.
2. Ajabnoor MA, Tilmisany AK. Effect of Trigonella foenum graceum on blood glucose levels in normal and alloxan-diabetic mice. *J Ethnopharmacol* 1988;22:45–49.
3. Khosla P, Gupta DD, Nagpal RK. Effect of Trigonella foenum graecum (Fenugreek) on blood glucose in normal and diabetic rats. *Indian J Physiol Pharmacol* 1995;39:173–174.
4. Ali L, Azad Khan AK, et al. Characterization of the hypoglycemic effects of Trigonella foenum graecum seed. *Planta Med* 1995;61:358–360.
5. Haefele C, Bonfils C, Sauvaire Y. Characterization of a dioxygenase from Trigonella foenum-graecum involved in 4-hyrdrox-yleucine biosynthesis. *Phytochemistry* 1997;44:563–566.
6. Sharma RD, Raghuram TC, Rao NS. Effect of fenugreek seeds on blood glucose and serum lipids in type I diabetes. *Eur J Clin Nutr* 1990;44:301–306.
7. Bordia A, Verma SK, Srivastava KC. Effect of ginger (Zingiber officinale Rosc.) and fenugreek (Trigonella foenumgraecum L.) on blood lipids, blood sugar and platelet aggre-gation in patients with coronary artery dis-

ease. *Prostaglandins Leukot Essent Fatty Acids* 1997;56:379–384.

8. Stark A, Madar Z. The effect of an ethanol extract derived from fenugreek (Trigonella foenum-graecum) on bile acid absorption and cholesterol levels in rats. *Br J Nutr* 1993;69:277–287.

9. Petit PR, Sauvaire YD, et al. Steroid saponins from fenugreek seeds: extraction, purification, and pharmacological investigation on feeding behavior and plasma cholesterol. *Steroids* 1995;60:674–680.

10. Ravikumar P, Anuradha CV. Effect of fenugreek seeds on blood lipid peroxidation and antioxidants in diabetic rats. *Phytother Res* 1999;13:197–201.

11. Javan M, Ahmadiani A, et al. Antinociceptive effects of Trigonella foenum-graecum leaves extract. *J Ethnopharmacol* 1997;58:125–129.

12. Yadav SK, Sehgal S. Effect of home processing and storage on ascorbic acid and beta-carotene content of Bathua (Chenopodium album) and fenugreek (Trigonella foenum graecum) leaves. *Planta Foods Hum Nutr* 1997;50:239–247.

13. Ahsan SK, Tariq M, et al. Effect of Trigonella foenum-graecum and Ammi majus on calcium oxalate urolithiasis in rats. *J Ethnopharmacol* 1989;26:249–254.

14. Patil SP, Niphadkar PV, Bapat MM. Allergy to fenugreek (Trigonella foenum graecum). *Ann Allergy Asthma Immunol* 1997;78:297–300.

*VALERIANA SP./*VALERIAN

1. Prabhu V, Karanath KS, Rao A. Effects of Nardostachys jatamansi on biogenic amines and inhibitory amino acids in the rat brain. *Planta Med* 1994;60:140–117.

2. Blumenthal M. EAPC files petitions for OTC drug use for valerian and ginger. *HerbalGram* 1995;35:19–20.

3. Lindahl O, Lindwall L. Double-blind study of a valerian preparation. *Pharmacol Biochem Behav* 1989;32:1065–1066.

4. Schulz H, Stolz C, Muller J. The effect of valerian extract on sleep polygraphy in poor sleepers: a pilot study. *Pharmacopsychiatry* 1994;27:146–151.

5. Leatherwood P, Chauffard F, et al. Aqueous extract of valerian root *(Valeriana officinalis)* improves sleep quality in man. *Pharmacol Biochem Behav* 1982;17:6541.

6. Leatherwood PD, Chauffard F. Quantifying the effects of mild sedatives. *J Psychiatr Res* 1982–83;17:115–122.

7. Sakamoto T, Mitani Y, Nakajima K. Psychotropic effects of Japanese valerian root extracts. *Chem Pharm Bull (Tokyo)* 1992;40:758–761.

8. Andreatini R, Leite JR. Effect of valeprotriates on the behavior of rats in the elevated plus-maze during diazepam withdrawal. *Eur J Pharmacol* 1994;260:233–235.

9. Rasmussen P. A role for phytotherapy in the treatment of benzodiazepine and opiate drug withdrawal (Part 1). *The European J Herbal Medicine* 1997;3:11–21.

10. Rucker G, Tautges J, et al. Isolation and pharacodynamic activity of the sesquiterpene valeranone from Nardostachys jatamansi DC. *Arzneimittelforschung* 1978;28:7–13.

11. Hazelhoff B, Malingre TM, Meijer DK. Antispasmodic effects of valeriana compounds: an in-vivo and in-vitro study on the guinea-pig ileum. *Arch Int Pharmacodyn Ther* 1982;257:274–287.

12. Dixit VP, Jain P, Joshi SC. Hypolipidaemic effects of Cucurma longa L and Nardostachys jata, amsi DC in triton-induced hyperlipidaemic rats. *Indian J Physiol Pharmacol* 1988;32:299–304.

13. Sarbhoy AK, Varshney JL, et al. Efficacy of some essential oils and their constituents on

few ubiquitous molds. *Zentralbl Bakteriol (Naturwiss)* 1978;133:723–725.

14. Balderer G, Borbely AA. Effect of valerian on human sleep. *Psychopharmacology (Berl)* 1985;87:406–409.

15. Willey LB, Mady SP, et al. Valerian overdose: a case report. *Vet Hum Toxicol* 1995;37:364–365.

16. Gerhard U, Linnenbrink N, et al. Vigilance-decreasing effects of 2 plant-derived sedatives. *Schweiz Rundsch Med Prax* 1996;85:473–481.

WITHANIA SOMNIFERA/ASHWAGANDHA

1. Dhuley JN. Effect of ashwagandha on lipid peroxidation in stress-induced animals. *J Ethnopharmacol* 1998;60:173–178.

2. Bhattacharya SK, Satyan KS, Ghosal S. Antioxidant activity of glycowithanolides from Withania somnifera. *Indian J Exp Biol* 1997;35:236–239.

3. Dhuley JN. Effect of some Indian herbs on macrophage functions in ochratoxin A treated mice. *J Ethnopharmacol* 1997;58:15–20.

4. Ziauddin M, Phansalkar N, et al. Studies on the immunomodulatory effects of Ashwagandha. *J Ethnopharmacol* 1996;50:69–76.

5. Kuttan G. Use of Withania somnifera Dunal as an adjuvant during radiation therapy. *Indian J Exp Biol* 1996;34:854–856.

6. Davis L, Kuttan G. Suppressive effect of cyclophosphamide-induced toxicity by Withania somnifera extract in mice. *J Ethnopharmacol* 1998;62:209–214.

7. Devi PU, Akagi K, et al. Withaferin A: a new radiosensitizer from the Indian medicinal plant Withania somnifera. *Int J Radiat Biol* 1996;69:193–197.

8. Mehta AK, Binkley P, et al. Pharmacological effects of Withania somnifera root extract on GABA receptor complex. *Indian J Med Res* 1991;94:312–315.

9. Schleibs R, Liebmann A, et al. Systemic administration of defined extracts from Witha-nia somnifera (Indian Ginseng) and Shilajit differentially affects cholinergic but not glutamatergic and GABAergic markers in rat brain. *Neurochem Int* 1997;30:181–190.

10. Karnick CR. A double-blind, placebo controlled clinical study on the effects of Withania somnifera and Panax ginseng extracts on psychomotor performance in healthy Indian volunteers. *Indian Med* 1991;3:1–5.

ZINGIBER OFFICINALE/GINGER

1. Phillips S, Ruggier R, Hutchinson SE. Zingiber officinale (ginger)—an antiemetic for day case surgery. *Anaesthesia* 1993;48:715–717.

2. Arfeen Z, Owen H, et al. A double-blind randomized controlled trial of ginger for the prevention of postoperative nausea and vomiting. *Anaesth Intensive Care* 1995;23:449–452.

3. Schmid R, Schick T, et al. Comparison of seven commonly used agents for prophylaxis of seasickness. *J Travel Med* 1994;1:203–206.

4. Mowrey DB, Clayson DE. Motion sickness, ginger and psychophysics. *The Lancet* 1982;1:655–657.

5. Fischer-Rasmussen W, Kjaer SK, et al. Ginger treatment of hyperemesis gravidarum. *Eur J Obstet Gynecol Reprod Ciol* 1991;38:19–24.

6. Fulder S, Tenne M. Ginger as an anti-nausea remedy in pregnancy—the issue of safety. *HerbalGram* 38:47–50.

7. Sharma SS, Gupta YK. Reversal of cisplatin-induced delay in gastric emptying in rats by ginger (Zingiber officinale). *J Ethnopharmacol* 1998;62:49–55.

8. Bhandari U, Sharma JN, Zafar R. The protective action of ethanolic ginger (Zingiber officinale) extract in cholesterol fed rabbits. *J Ethnopharmacol* 1998;61:167–171.

9. Verma SK, Singh J, et al. Effect of ginger on platelet aggregation in man. *Indian J Med Res* 1993;98:240–242.

THE CHOPRA CENTER HERBAL FORMULARY SUPPORT FORMULAS

Many of the herbs described in this book are available as components of the Chopra Center Herbal Formulary Support formulas. For more information on these and other nutritional supplements, visit our website at www.MyPotential.com

The Forty Herbs of the Chopra Formulary

Latin Name	Circulation	Detox	Digestion	Immune	Prostate	Metabolism	Mind	Energy	Sleep	Menopause
Allium sativum										
Aloe vera										
Andrographis paniculata				X						
Asparagus racemosus								X		X
Astragalus membraneceus				X						
Azadirachta indica		X								
Boswellia serrata										
Camellia sinensis	X							X		
Cassia angustifolia										
Centella asiatica/ Bacopa monniera	X						X	X		
Cimicifuga racemosa										X
Coleus forskohlii	X									
Commiphora mukul	X					X				
Crataegus oxyacantha	X									
Curcurma longa										
Echinacea purpurea				X						
Eletteria cardamomum			X							
Emblica officinalis		X	X		X	X		X		X
Ginkgo biloba							X			
Glycyrrhiza glabra										X

The Forty Herbs of the Chopra Formulary

Latin Name	Circulation	Detox	Digestion	Immune	Prostate	Metabolism	Mind	Energy	Sleep	Menopause
Gymnema syvlestre						X				
Hypericum perforatum										
Lavandula angustifolia										
Linum usitatissimum										
Melaleuca alternifolia										
Mucuna pruriens					X					
Ocimum sanctum										
Phyllanthus niruri		X								
Picrorhiza kurroa		X				X				
Piper methysticum										
Serenoa repens					X					
Silybum marianum		X								
Tanacetum parthenium										
Terminalia arjuna	X									
Tinospora cordifolia				X						
Trigonella foenum-graecum										
Ulmus fulva										
Valeriana									X	
Withania somnifera	X			X	X		X	X		
Zingiber officinale			X			X				

RECOMMENDED HERBAL REFERENCES

Blumenthal, Mark. *The Complete German Commission E Monographs.* Boston, Mass.: American Botanical Council, 1998.

Chevallier, Andrew. *The Encyclopedia of Medicinal Plants.* London: Dorling Kindersley Limited, 1996.

Dash, Bhagwan. *Materia Medica of Ayurveda.* New Delhi: B. Jain Publishers, 1991.

Dastur, J. F. *Medicinal Plants of India and Pakistan.* Bombay: D. B. Taraporevala Sons & Co., 1962.

Dutt, U. C. *Materia Medica of the Hindus.* Calcutta: Krinshnadas Sanskrit Studies, 1922.

Kapoor, L. D. *Handbook of Ayurvedic Medicinal Plants.* Boca Raton: CRC Press, 1990.

Lad, Vasant, and David Frawley. 1986. *The Yoga of Herbs.* Santa Fe: Lotus Press, 1986.

Mowrey, Daniel B. *The Scientific Validation of Herbal Medicine.* New Canaan, Conn.: Keats Publishing, 1986.

Patnaik, Naveen. *The Garden of Life.* New York: Doubleday, 1993.

Pizzorno, Joseph E., and Murray, Michael T. *A Textbook of Natural Medicine.* Bothell, Wash.: Bastyr University Publications, 1996.

Tierra, Michael. *Planetary Herbology.* Santa Fe: Lotus Press, 1988.

Tyler, Varro E. *The Honest Herbal.* New York: Pharmaceutical Products Press, 1993.

RECOMMENDED AYURVEDIC REFERENCES

Chopra, Deepak. *Perfect Health*. New York: Harmony Books, 2000.

Dash, Bhagwan. *A Handbook of Ayurveda*. New Delhi: Concept Publishing, 1987.

Frawley, David. *Ayurvedic Healing*. Salt Lake City: Passage Press, 1989.

Joshi, Sunil. *Ayurveda & Panchakarma*. Twin Lakes, Wisc.: Lotus Press, 1996.

Renade, Subash. *Natural Healing Through Ayurveda*. Salt Lake City: Passage Press, 1993.

Simon, David. *The Wisdom of Healing*. Rider Books, 1997.

INDEX

NOTE: Bold page numbers refer to primary discussions of topic.

Blood pressure
  and arjuna, 184
  and black cohosh, 99
  and coleus, 101, 102, 103, 104
  and ephedrine, 42
  and garlic, 63, 64, 65
  and hawthorn, 50, 109
  and holy basil, 160
  and Indian gentian, 71
  and licorice, 131, 132, 133
  and phyllanthus, 164
  precautions concerning, 104, 133
  and senna, 90
  and snakeroot, 49
  and tea, 88
  and valerian, 198
Blood sugar, 81, 99, 162, 164, 184,
    187, 189, 190. *See also*
    Diabetes
Blood thinning, 65, 89, 106, 107,
    114, 129, 182, 206, 210
Boswellia, 45, 56, 58, 59, 60, **83–86**
Bowel disorders, 16, 67, 75, 83, 88,
    122, 124, 194
Bowel movements. *See* Diarrhea;
    Elimination; Laxatives
Brahmi. *See* Gotu kola
Breast cancer, 64, 88
Breastfeeding, 73, 74, 75, 93, 111,
    168, 176, 191
Breath freshener, 121, 145
Bronchitis, 132, 168, 195
Burns, 66, 68, 145, 151–52, 194, 195

C
Calming herbs, 22, 28, **39–40**, 210.
    See also specific herb
Camphor, 11, 22, 28, 45
Cancer, 11, 35, 36, 47, 48
  and aloe vera, 67
  and *amrit*, 187, 188
  and arjuna, 184
  and astragalus, 76, 77–78
  and coleus, 103
  and echinacea, 116, 117
  and garlic, 62, 63–64
  and gotu kola, 95
  and holy basil, 158
  and Indian gooseberry, 123
  and licorice, 131

  and St. John's wort, 140
  and senna, 91
  and slippery elm, 195
  and tea, 87–88
  and turmeric, 112, 113
  and winter cherry, 202
  See also Chemotherapy; *type of
    cancer*
Candida, 74, 151, 152
Canker sores, 106, 132
Capsaicin, 45
Cardamom, 18, 21, 22, 37, 38, 56,
    58, 60, 88, 113, **119–21**
Cardiovascular system, 50, 62, 63,
    87, 90, 102, 108, 109,
    112, 183, 184. *See also* Heart dis-
    ease
Cascara sagrada, 16, 38, 68, 91
Castor oil, 38, 91
Cayenne, 17, 18, 28, 37
Cedarwood, 144–45
Celery seeds, 37
Chamomile, 20–21, 22, 37, 45, 96,
    113
Charaka school, 25–26
Charts
  about names of herbs, 58–61
  about uses for herbs, 56–57
Chaste-tree berries, 40
Chavan Prash jam, 123–24, 208
Chemotherapy, 46, 81, 120, 159, 161,
    178, 187, 195, 201, 204
Childbirth/labor, 40, 91, 97, 99, 144,
    194
Chili peppers, 45
Cholesterol
  and *amrit*, 187
  and arjuna, 50, 183, 184
  and cowage plant, 156
  and fenugreek, 189–90, 191
  and flaxseed, 147–48
  and garlic, 63, 64
  and ginger, 204
  and gum gugal, 43, 105, 106, 107
  and gurmar, 135
  and hawthorn, 109
  and holy basil, 160
  and Indian gentian, 71
  and Indian gooseberry, 123, 124
  and licorice, 131

  and milk thistle, 177
  precautions concerning, 124
  and senna, 92
  and tea, 88
  and turmeric, 112
  and valerian, 197
Chondroitin sulfates, 45
Chronic disorders, 25, 35, 36, 47, 82.
    See also specific disorder
  Chronic fatigue syndrome, 67,
    117, 132, 163
Cinnamon, 17, 18, 20, 22, 28, 37–38,
    114, 195
Circulation, **49–50**
  and arjuna, 183, 186
  and astragalus, 78, 79
  and boswellia, 86
  and cardamom, 120, 121
  chart of herbs for, 56–57
  and coleus, 103, 104
  and flaxseed, 149
  and garlic, 49–50, 65
  and ginger, 204, 205, 206
  and ginkgo, 125, 126, 127, 129
  and gum gugal, 49–50, 105, 107
  and hawthorn, 50, 108, 109, 111
  and holy basil, 161
  and Indian gentian, 70, 71, 73
  and Indian gooseberry, 124
  and licorice, 133
  and picroliv, 169
  and slippery elm, 196
  and tea, 89
Clotting, 50, 84, 106, 123, 129, 131,
    156
Clove, 17, 18, 20, 28, 47, 88, 121
Coconut oil, 22
Cold sores, 194
Colds
  and *amrit*, 188
  and astragalus, 78
  and cardamom, 120
  and chamomile, 113
  and cinnamon, 114
  and coriander, 114
  and echinacea, 46, 117
  and fenugreek, 191
  and ginger, 205
  and holy basil, 158, 160
  and Indian gentian, 71, 72

Epstein-Barr virus, 163
Eyes, 22, 102, 194

F

Fatigue, 36, 39, 47
  and cardamom, 121
  and cloves, 121
  and echinacea, 117
  and hawthorn, 110
  and picroliv, 168
  and St. John's wort, 142
  and tea, 87, 121
  and winter cherry, 201
  See also Chronic fatigue syndrome
Fennel, 18, 28, 37, 38, 121, 124
Fenugreek, 17, 57, 59, 60, 113, **189–92**
Fertility, 73, 75, 78, 154, 156, 161, 173, 175, 202
Fever, 47, 71, 80, 96, 114, 131, 137, 164, 168
Feverfew, 4, 16, 45, 50, 57, 59, 60, **179–82**
Fibromyalgia, 107
Fire, as element, 26, 28, 30–31, 32, 36–37
Flaxseed, 21, 38, 57, 59, 60, 92, **146–49**
Flu, 72, 78, 113, 114, 117, 120, 158, 160, 188
Food, 16–18, 49. *See also* Appetite; Digestion; Eating
Forskolin. *See* Coleus
Foxglove, 8, 49

G

Gallbladder/gallstones, 113, 167, 185
Garcinia cambogia, 42
Garlic, 21, 49–50, 56, 58, 60, **62–65**
Gas/gastritis, 18, 28, 37, 38, 85, 105, 120, 145, 158
Gentian. *See* Indian gentian
Ginger, **203–6**
  and Ayurveda principles, 205, 206
  botanical and phytochemical information about, 203–4
  and elements of plants, 28
  and herbal energetics, 32

  and history of herbal medicine, 10
  how to use, 205
  names for, 59, 60, 203
  and other herbs, 88, 113, 121, 132
  precautions concerning, 206
  science of, 204
  side effects of, 203
  taste of, 18, 203
  uses for, 18, 20, 22, 37, 40, 42, 47, 57, 113, 121, 132, 203, 204–5, 206
Ginkgo, 11, 28, 40, 56, 60, **125–29**
Ginseng, 10, 187
  uses for, 21, 40, 43, 48, 49, 71, 200, 201, 208
Glaucoma, 102
Gokshura, 44, 175
Goldenseal, 10, 20, 37, 46, 118
Gonorrhea, 85, 184
Gotu kola, 28, 39, 40, 56, 58, 60, **94–97**, 168, 208
Gout, 188, 194
Green tea, 18, 87, 88, 89, 109
Guggulu. *See* Gum gugal
Gum gugal, **104–7**
  and Ayurveda principles, 107
  botanical and phytochemical information about, 105
  as calming herb, 39
  dosage of, 107
  as heating herb, 107
  how to use, 107, 209
  names for, 58, 60, 104
  and other herbs, 107, 124, 184
  precautions concerning, 107
  science of, 105–6
  side effects of, 105
  tastes of, 107
  uses for, 39, 42–43, 45, 49–50, 56, 104, 106–7, 124, 184, 209
Gurmar, 57, 59, 60, **134–37**

H

Hair loss, 145
Hallucinogenics, 28
Haridra. *See* Turmeric
Haritaki, 38, 42
Hawthorn, 50, 56, 58, 60, **108–11**
Headaches, 45, 96, 97, 105, 129, 142, 145, 198, 205. *See also* Migraine headaches

Health
  characteristics of good, 3
  definition of, 27, 214
  disease as absence of, 36
  and elements of plants, 27
  as state of dynamic balance, 33
Health problems, three issues for considering, 29
Hearing, 22, 125, 127, 128
Heart disease, 8, 35, 47
  and arjuna, 50, 185
  and astragalus, 78
  and black cohosh, 99
  and coleus, 101, 102
  and garlic, 63
  and gum gugal, 106
  and hawthorn, 50, 109–10, 111
  and holy basil, 159
  and Indian gentian, 71
  and Indian gooseberry, 48, 123, 124
  and licorice, 131
  precautions concerning, 111
  and tea, 88
  and turmeric, 112
  See also Cardiovascular system
Heart rhythm/irregularities, 4, 109, 110, 198
Heartburn, 18, 28, 37
  and aloe vera, 68
  and boswellia, 85
  and ginger, 206
  and holy basil, 160
  and Indian gooseberry, 16, 37, 75, 123, 132
  and licorice, 16, 37, 75, 132
  and slippery elm, 194
  and wild asparagus, 37, 74, 132
Helicobacter pylori, 64
Hemorrhoids, 193, 194
Hepatitis, 68, 131, 162, 163, 164, 167, 168, 177, 178
Herbal renaissance, 1–5
Herbs/herbal medicine
  as alternative medicine, 2
  appropriate use of, 32–33
  and benefits of taking several herbs together, 209–10
  charts about, 56–61

Space, as element, 26, 28, 30–31, 32
Stomach ailments, 100, 120, 124, 145, 195
Stomach cancer, 64
Stress, 48–49
    and *amrit*, 187–88
    and ginseng, 187
    and gum gugal, 106
    and hawthorn, 110
    and holy basil, 159, 160
    and lavender, 144
    and turmeric, 112
    and valerian, 197, 198
    and winder cherry, 201
    and winter cherry, 187
Strokes, 50, 106, 171
Sunburn, 195
Sunflower oil, 22
Suppositories, 194
Surgery, 91, 95, 96, 128, 187, 204
Sweet basil, 161
Swelling/bloating, 18, 29, 37, 38
    and aloe vera, 68
    and basil, 38, 158, 160
    and cardamom, 18, 120
    and gotu kola, 95
    and gum gugal, 105, 106
Syphilis, 85, 188

T
Tastes, **16–18**, 19, 31–33, 43. *See also specific taste or herb*
Tea, 56, 58, 61, **86–89**, 109. *See also type of tea*
Tea tree, 57, 59, 61, **150–53**
Thyme, 17, 18, 28, 38, 45, 144–45
Tonsillitis, 71
Touch, 22
Tranquilizers, 169, 170–71. *See also* Calming herbs; Sedatives
Triglycerides, 43, 105, 106, 160, 190
Trikatu, 42
Trimada, 42
Triphala formula, 21, 38, 42, 107, 122, 124, 132
Tuberculosis, 167
Turmeric, **111–14**
    and Ayurveda principles, 114
    botanical and phytochemical information about, 112

as heating herb, 114
how to use, 113–14
names for, 58, 61, 111
and other herbs, 68, 81, 84, 113, 114, 168
precautions concerning, 114
science of, 112–13
side effects of, 112
taste of, 113, 114
uses for, 45, 45, 47, 50, 56, 68, 111, 113, 114, 124

U
Ulcers, 37, 195
    and aloe vera, 68
    and arjuna, 185
    and boswellia, 84, 85
    and cardamom, 121
    and garlic, 64
    and ginkgo, 128
    and gotu kola, 95
    and holy basil, 160
    and licorice, 37, 131–32
    and neem, 81
    precautions concerning, 85, 121
    and slippery elm, 194
    and turmeric, 112
    and valerian, 197
    and winter cherry, 202
Urinary tract
    and *amrit*, 75
    and boswellia, 84
    and flaxseed, 147
    and hawthorn, 108
    and herbs for men's health, 44
    and Indian gentian, 71
    and phyllanthus, 163, 164
    and saw palmetto, 173, 174–75
    and slippery elm, 194
    and wild asparagus, 75
U.S. Food and Drug Administration (FDA), 12
Uterus, 74

V
Vajikarana herbs, 43
Valerian, 16, 20–21, 39, 57, 59, 61, 96, **196–99**
Varicose veins, 138

Vata principle, 28, 29, 30–31
    See also specific herb
Vidanga, 42
Vitex agnuscastus, 41

W
Walnuts, 49
Water, as element, 26–28, 29, 32
Weight, 29, 36, 43
    and boswellia, 85
    and fenugreek, 190
    and ginger, 206
    and gum gugal, 42–43, 105, 106
    and gurmar, 136–37
    and licorice, 132
    and neem, 80, 81, 82
    and tea, 88
    and wild asparagus, 75
    See also Metabolism
Wholeness, herbs and, 22–23
Wild asparagus, **73–76**
    and Ayurveda principles, 75
    botanical and phytochemical information about, 74
    as cooling herb, 74–75
    and elements of plants, 27
    how to use, 75
    names for, 58, 61, 73
    and other herbs, 75, 124, 132, 156, 188
    precautions concerning, 75
    science of, 74
    taste of, 75
    uses for, 21, 37, 41, 46–47, 56, 73, 74–75, 76, 124, 132, 156, 188, 208
Wild buckwheat, 27
Wild celery seeds, 38
Willow tree bark, 44
Wind-pacifying herbs, 39
Winter cherry, 21, 27, 187, **200–202**
    and Ayurveda principles, 202
    botanical and phytochemical information about, 200–201
    how to use, 202
    names for, 59, 61, 200
    and other herbs, 84, 156, 188
    precautions concerning, 202
    science of, 201
    uses for, 43, 46, 48, 49, 57, 156, 188, 200, 201–2, 208

I n d e x   259

Deepak Chopra and The Chopra Center for Well Being in La Jolla, California, offer a wide range of seminars, products and educational programmes, worldwide. The Chopra Center offers revitalizing mind/body programmes, as well as day spa services. Guests can come to rejuvenate, expand knowledge or obtain a medical consultation.

For information on meditation classes, health and well-being courses, instructor certification programmes, or local classes in your area, contact The Chopra Center for Well Being, 7630 Fay Avenue, La Jolla, California 92037, U.S.A. By telephone: 001-888-424-6772, or 001-619-551-7788. For a virtual tour of the Center, visit the Internet website at www.chopra.com.

If you live in Europe and would like more information on workshops, lectures or other programmes about Dr. Deepak Chopra or to order any of his books, tapes or products, please contact: Contours, 44 Fordbridge Road, Ashford, Middlesex, TW15 2SJ (tel: +44 (0) 208 564 7033; fax: +44 (0) 208 897 3807; email: sales@infinite-contours.co.uk; website: www.infinite-contours.co.uk).

If you have enjoyed this book and would like the opportunity to explore higher realms of consciousness and have a more direct experience of divinity, you may do so interactively at Deepak Chopra's new website, www.mypotential.com.